Metformin - A Prospective Alternative for the Treatment of Chronic Diseases

Edited by Farid A. Badria

Published in London, United Kingdom

Metformin - A Prospective Alternative for the Treatment of Chronic Diseases
http://dx.doi.org/10.5772/intechopen.104352
Edited by Farid A. Badria

Contributors
Farid A. Badria, Ahmed R. Ali, Yhiya Amen, Adel F. Badria, Ahmed Elbermawi, Dario Rahelić, Zrinka Šakić, Eloy A. Zepeda-Carrillo, Rafael Torres Valadez, Sara A. Campos-Huerta, Elisa María Barrón Cabrera, Hongmei Tan, Jun Tao, Shafaat Husain Talib, Sachin Patel, Pranita Barapatre, Umar Quadri

First published in London, United Kingdom, 2023 by IntechOpen
IntechOpen is the global imprint of INTECHOPEN LIMITED, registered in England and Wales, registration number: 11086078, 5 Princes Gate Court, London, SW7 2QJ, United Kingdom

British Library Cataloguing-in-Publication Data
A catalogue record for this book is available from the British Library

Additional hard and PDF copies can be obtained from orders@intechopen.com

Metformin - A Prospective Alternative for the Treatment of Chronic Diseases
Edited by Farid A. Badria
p. cm.
Print ISBN 978-1-83768-238-6
Online ISBN 978-1-83768-239-3
eBook (PDF) ISBN 978-1-83768-240-9

Meet the editor

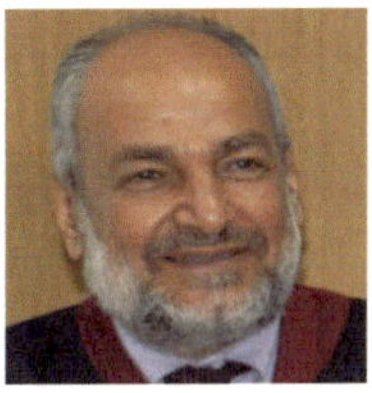

Professor Farid Badria, Ph.D., DSc, leads research projects on developing new therapies for liver, skin disorders, and cancer. He was among the top 2% of the most-cited scientists in medicinal and biomolecular chemistry in 2019, 2020, and 2021, according to the lists published by Stanford University, USA. He has been a scholar with the Arab Development Fund, Kuwait, ICRO-UNESCO, Chile, and UNESCO Biotechnology, France. Among the awards he has received are the TWAS Prize for the Public Understanding of Science, the WIPO Gold Medal for the best inventor, the State Outstanding Award in Medicine, the Outstanding Arab Scholar, Kuwait, and the Khawrazmi International Award, Iran. Prof. Badria has over 270 publications, including twelve books, has submitted 49 patents, 20 of which have received final certification, and has marketed several pharmaceutical products.

Contents

Preface

It is now known that the causes and pathogenesis of many complex chronic diseases are usually polyfactorial: genetic, environmental, constitutive factors, or a combination of these. Many compounds have emerged as new potential therapeutic drugs for the treatment of chronic and/or complex diseases.

Poly-target molecules have recently been recognized and efficiently used in the treatment of several metabolic disorders, infectious and inflammatory diseases. Enzymes capable of catalyzing several reactions are known as promiscuous enzymes, for example, lipase, which is capable of converting lipids, phospholipids or triglycerides into the corresponding fatty acids and alcohols. Promiscuity with respect to the substrate (e.g., an aryl esterase of carboxylic acids acting on an amide bond) can be called catalytic promiscuity. A further class of promiscuity is based on the capability of small molecules (e.g., valproate, metformin, aspirin, quinine) to selectively react with many receptors, leading to diverse pharmacological activities.

A combination of different pharmacophores can be chosen from single-target ligands and a series of compounds screened using computational models and/or optimization using *in vitro* assays. Computer-aided drug design (CADD) can be used to examine the possible interaction of ligand (drug) and receptor (target). Proteins/antigens, as found in many infectious diseases or cancers, must be carefully selected. Homologous proteins should not be present both in the causative agent and in the host.

This book discusses the diverse applications of multi-target compounds in the treatment of many chronic complex health disorders. Each chapter presents up-to-date poly-pharmacology research, with particular reference to metformin, the broad-ranging applications of which are illustrated in the circle below.

Chapter 1 presents the chemical and biological poly-pharmacology of metformin. New insights into the use of metformin for diabetic patients are introduced in Chapter 2. Chapter 3 reviews the beneficial effects of metformin on DM-related cardiovascular complications and dissects the potential molecular mechanisms. while Chapter 4 discusses glycemic and extraglycemic effects of metformin in patients with diabetes. Chapter 5 familiarizes the effects of metformin in non-diabetes related medical disorders, advances in our understanding of this drug and its pathways in health and diseases.

We hope this book will be useful to a wide range of readers, from students first learning about natural coloring compounds, to advanced clinicians, nutrition specialists, and researchers looking for a review of current treatments and conceptualizations of chronic conditions.

Farid A. Badria
FAB-Lab,
Faculty of Pharmacy,
Pharmacognosy Department,
Mansoura University,
Mansoura, Egypt

Section 1

Introduction to Metformin

Chapter 1

Metformin: A Small Molecule with Multi-Targets and Diverse Therapeutic Applications

Farid A. Badria, Ahmed R. Ali, Ahmed Elbermawi, Yhiya Amen and Adel F. Badria

Abstract

Metformin is one of the most prescribed agents in the treatment of type 2 diabetes. Its history goes back to the use of goat's rue (*Galega officinalis* Linn., Fabaceae). *G. officinalis* is rich in galegine, a guanidine derivative with a blood glucose-lowering effect. Research based on the effects of guanidine rich on this traditional herbal medicine led to the development of metformin. Metformin continues to serve as a multi-target drug. Its benefits for treating/controlling several diseases were thoroughly discovered over time. These include health disorders such as cancers, obesity, periodontitis, cardiovascular, liver, skin, and renal disorders. Moreover, there is evidence to propose that metformin postpones the aging processes as well as modulates the microbiota to promote better health. So far, it is not fully understood, how metformin can accomplish such pleiotropic pharmacological and therapeutic effects. Metformin may decrease malignancy via suppressing the signal of insulin/IGF-1, avoiding the release of cytokines via NF-κB, and increasing the immune reaction to cancer cells. This chapter discusses the history of metformin discovery, chemistry, its role in diabetic patients, and proposed molecular mechanisms to shed more light on the diverse effects and its ability to target multiple signaling pathways.

Keywords: metformin, galegine, biguanides, type 2 diabetes, drug repurposing, cancer, metabolic disorders, degenerative diseases

1. Introduction

Currently, polyfunctional or polypharmacy or multiple targets may present new therapeutic avenues for drugs for the treatment of many chronic and/or complex health disorders which constitute multifactorial pathogenesis, for example, genetics, environment, and lifestyle.

Recently, poly-target molecules including metformin have been recognized and efficiently used in the treatment of several metabolic disorders, infectious, and inflammatory diseases.

2. Concept of multi-target drugs

Polyfunction or polypharmacy or multiple targets have emerged as new potential therapeutic drugs for the treatment of chronic and/or complex diseases. It is well-known that many chronic diseases are usually polyfactorial including different genetics, environment, constitutive, and mixed aspects [1].

Recently, poly-target molecules have been recognized and efficiently used in the treatment of several metabolic disorders, infectious, and inflammatory diseases [1]. Promiscuous enzyme is an enzyme that is capable to catalyze several reactions; for example, lipase enzyme is capable to convert lipids or phospholipids or triglycerides to corresponding fatty acids and alcohols [2]. Also, the promiscuity of substrate (aryl esterase of carboxylic acids) acts on amide bond and could be called catalytic promiscuity. Moreover, there is another class of promiscuity based on the capability of small molecules (e.g., valproate, aspirin, and quinine) to selectively react with many receptors leading to diverse pharmacological activities [2].

Acetylsalicylic acid proved to act by different physiological and pharmacological targets; for example, cyclooxygenase enzyme which may modulate several signaling pathways, and subsequently prompt poly-target-dependent pharmacological activities [1].

3. Approaches for developing multi-targets agents

3.1 Approach 1 (fragment-based)

Choosing a combination of different pharmacophores from single-target ligands and screening a series of compounds using several computational models and/or via optimizing in vitro assays [3].

3.2 Approach 2 (selection-based target)

Based upon the selection of preferentially expressed protein/antigen as manifested in many infectious diseases or cancer. These selected proteins must not retain homologous proteins in the same person or the selected proteins ought to be different to keep the selectivity [1, 3]. However, in this approach many other parameters need to be considered:

1. The characteristics of the disease under investigation (inflammatory, infectious, metabolic, or complex).

2. The mode of drug/compound resistance (adaptive or mutation or amplification of target amplification) [1].

3.3 Approach 3 (molecular docking or computer-assisted drug [CAD])

The design of CAD may be used to examine the possible ligand (drug) interaction with a receptor (target) to figure out the existing energy and possible extent of interaction. Therefore, based on this approach, we may arrange the existent ligand–target interactions based on the calculated energy. The prediction of interaction will be based on binding energy between a drug/compound and a target [4].

4. Applications of multi-targets compounds

4.1 Complex health disorders (CHDs)

Several inherent and/or environmental factors represent the major causes of the complex health disorders as presented in **Figure 1**. There are many examples of CHDs but not limited to malignancy.

4.2 Drug resistance

Drug resistance may be defined as a decrease in the efficacy of certain drugs; for example, anticancer, antimicrobial, and anti-epilepsy in curing or alleviating the symptoms and/or conditions of a certain disease. Moreover, the term "drug resistance" could be used alternatively in acquiring resistance to many types of cancers or common pathogens.

Generally, drug resistance may be attributed to one or more of the following mechanisms [1–4]:

- Releasing of drug/compound-inactivating enzymes
- Alteration of an existing receptor
- Acquisition of a site/target by-pass system
- Reduction of permeability of cells

The activity of metformin on modulating drug resistance of several types of cancers may influence the proliferation and metastasis of resistant cells resistant to

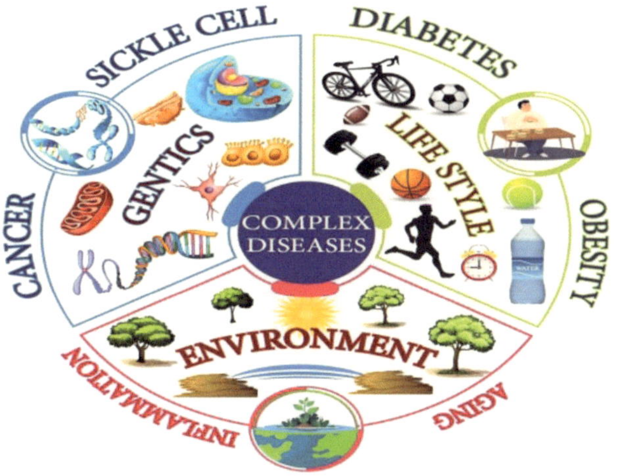

Figure 1.
Complex health disorders (CHDs) may present complex and combined factors; for example, genetics, environment, and lifestyle which may represent the major causes of complex health disorders, metabolic disorders, chronic degenerative, inflammatory, and neurological disorders. Multi-target compounds are very much valuable in the modulation of CHDs where patients may avoid the risk of drug–drug interaction, drug intolerance, and sustain better tolerance and pharmacokinetics [4].

tamoxifen or paclitaxel in the case of breast cancer, for example, via focusing on many changes in the Scribble (SCRIB)-induced activation of the Hippo pathway [5].

Metformin (MET), which exhibits anti-cancer activity via induction of AMP-activated protein kinase (AMPK), directly phosphorylates YAP and inhibits YAP transcriptional activity [6, 7].

4.3 Drug repositioning

Drug discovery or development of new drugs can be very lasting, costly, prone to many side effects, tolerability, and toxicity, as well as high cost [8]. Therefore, drug repositioning or drug repurposing may consider a well-accepted concept. For the last decade, metformin has been extensively proven high safety and tolerability in many clinical trials, especially when used as adjuvant therapy in many resistant drug cancer [8].

Drug repurposing may include a broad spectrum of old or recently approved drugs; for example, FDA-approved drugs or old, or even shelved drugs. Serendipity was the main avenue for discovering new uses for commonly available old drugs. However, computer-assisted drugs (CAD) showed to be an efficient method for retrospectively discovering new uses/targets for several known drugs [9].

5. Metformin: a unique model for small molecules with multi-target effects

Metformin molecules retained unique chemical and dynamic features. Chemically, metformin is a derivative of guanidine, one of the closely related active components in *Galega officinalis* Linn. (goat's rue) [9]. Chemical studies of *G. officinalis* showed that the plant was rich in guanidine and related compounds and proved to have hypoglycemic activity in animals but retained high toxicity in humans [10]. Therefore, a less toxic component of *G. officinalis*, galegine (isoamylguanidine), has been brought

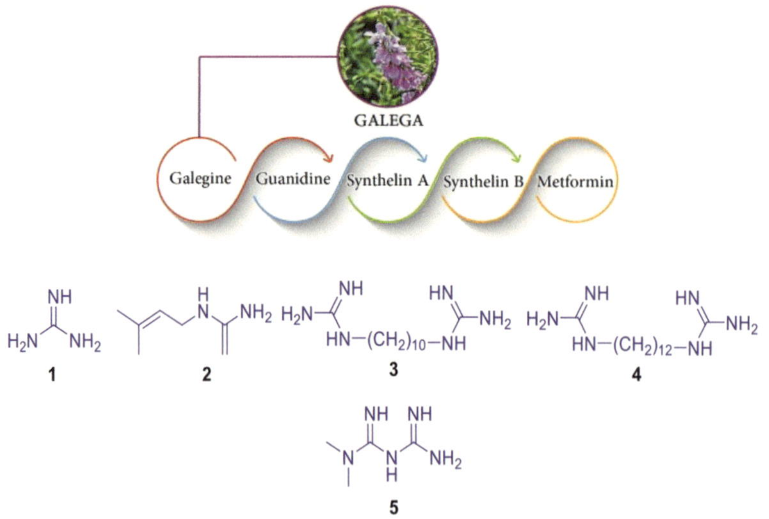

Figure 2.
Evolution of metformin discovery from Galega officinalis plant; guanidine (1), galegine (2), synthelin A (3), synthelin B (4), and metformin (5).

to light and it was used as an antidiabetic agent in the 1920s. Unfortunately, its toxicity caused it to be swiftly discontinued. However, the unique chemical nature of galegine has led the pharmaceutical industry to a new drug lead with lipophilic nature [11]; for example, Synthelin A (decamethylene diguanide) and Synthelin B (dodecamethylene diguanide) with better activity, tolerability, and unique dynamic and energetic structure as well as the interaction features with DNA minor grooves with AT-rich minor grooves of DNA [11–14] (**Figure 2**).

Generally, metformin, a biguanide derivate, is considered a safe drug. However, the evolution for developing metformin starts from galagine (1) which was isolated from *G. officinalis* plant, then followed by guanidine (2), biguanidine with (-CH2-)10 chain, (-CH2-)12 chains as a linker between the two guanidine moieties for Synthalin A (3) and Synthalin B (4), respectively. Unfortunately, even though their antihyperglycemic activity was better than metformin but showed to be more toxic with several side effects.

6. Metformin uses in CHDs

There are diverse and multiple therapeutic targets; inflammation, metabolic disorders, cancer, and degenerative diseases which are revealed to be hit by metformin as presented in **Figure 3**.

6.1 Metabolic disorders

This may include type 2 diabetes (DM-Type II), obesity, atherosclerosis (CVDs, NASH), inflammation, and infectious disorders.

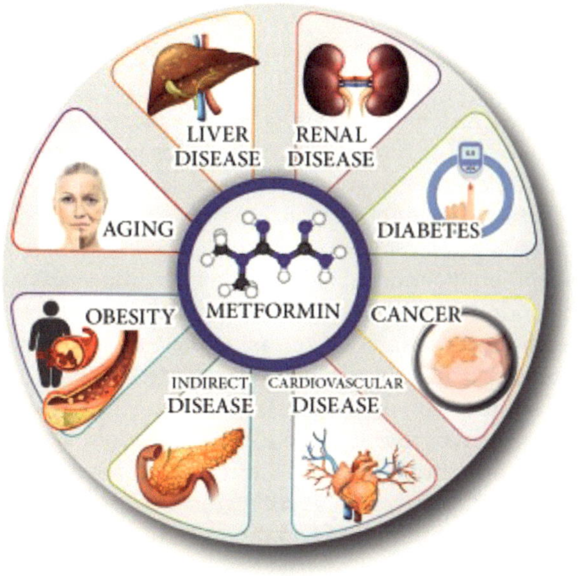

Figure 3.
Metformin has been recognized and efficiently used in the treatment of several metabolic disorders, infectious, and inflammatory diseases. Having an enzyme capable to catalyze several reactions (Promiscuous enzyme); for example, lipase enzyme is capable to convert lipids or phospholipids or triglycerides to corresponding fatty acids and alcohols.

6.1.1 Hepatic gluconeogenesis

Metformin can regulate hepatic gluconeogenesis via different mechanisms; for example, activation of AMPK which leads to accumulation of AMP and subsequently reduces the level of cAMP via inhibition of adenylate cyclase. Moreover, glycerophosphate dehydrogenase (mGPD) in mitochondria (enzyme responsible for converting glycerol to dihydroxyacetone phosphate). This inhibitory activity of mGPD will lead to the augmentation of both glycerol and glycerol-3-phosphate and suppress glucogenesis via alteration of the redox state in the cytosol [15].

6.1.2 Gut microbiome and inflammation

The gastrointestinal (GIT) physiology with its gut microbiota in glucose metabolism plays a major role in metformin efficacy and tolerance. Healthy GIT may contain huge numbers of microorganisms not limited to bacteria and fungi but may have viruses, protozoa, and fungi. The collective microbiome genomes encode over 100-fold genes more than the human genome generating many metabolites which can affect the health of the human; for example, inflammation, immunity, and microenvironment metabolism as production of fatty acid (short-chain fatty acid [SCFA]) which may lead to type 2 diabetes [16]. Therefore, a clinical study proved the capability of metformin to increase the number of beneficial bacteria such as *E. coli* species which proved to reduce the risk of the incidence of type 2 diabetes. On the other hand, the role of the microbiome as a cause or result for therapeutic benefit would require further investigation [17].

Metformin multi-targeted actions are induced through non-AMPK pathways and AMPK mechanisms [18]. Therefore, a wide range of beneficial effects were observed in several systems of the body including GIT, lung, kidney, pancreas, and CVS [18].

6.1.3 Cardiovascular systems

A prospective study carried out in the UK (UKPDS) showed that cardiovascular diseases are a major complication of type 2 diabetes [19]. Separately, in the USA the program for the prevention of type 2 diabetes revealed the significant role of metformin in the prevention of type 2 diabetes via its effects on impaired glucose tolerance (IGT) [20].

Metformin has shown positive progress in the number of clinical outcomes of CVD, including dyslipidemia, endothelial dysfunction, and systemic inflammation [21]. Regarding endothelial dysfunction, Metformin does this improvement by increasing nitric oxide synthase (eNOS) releasing the vasodilator agent, nitric oxide (NO). Additional pathways include stimulation of AMPK, inhibition of mitochondrial complex 1, and suppression of apoptosis [22].

Metformin has shown favorable effects on blood flow in several studies. It was able to enhance the reaction of hemodynamics to amino acid L-arginine (early NO precursor, vasodilator agent) [23]. Metformin also decreased dimethylarginine levels (NOS endogenous inhibitor) and reduce clot formation via diminishing platelet activity reduced through extracellular mitochondrial DNA (mtDNA) release [24].

6.1.4 Inflammation and infection

Metformin was initially used in many infectious diseases; for example, influenza and as a synergetic drug treatment in broad numbers of common diseases [25].

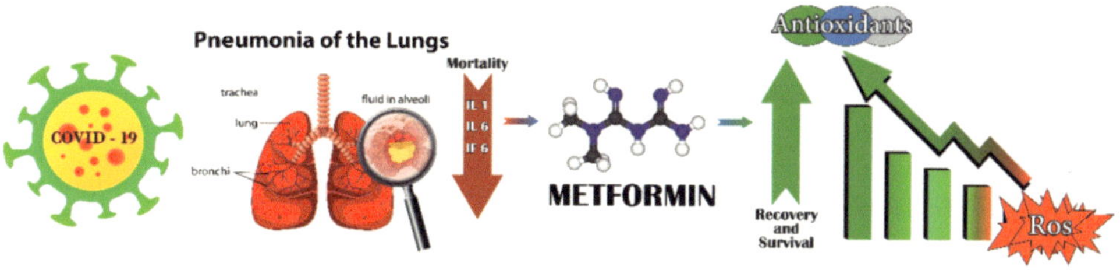

Figure 4.
Metformin with unique chemical features, multiple therapeutic targets, high safety therapeutic margin, and affordable economic cost may contribute to reducing mortality and improving recovery due to pandemic diseases; for example, COVID-19 and its fatal complications.

Repurposing metformin for fighting the current pandemic of COVID-19 represented a promising strategy as an adjunctive therapy by altering the immune responses to treat infections [26, 27]. A great advantage of metformin use is its lower mortality rate in patients with type 2 diabetes affected by COVID-19 when compared to its counterparts, especially among women population with obesity [28, 29]. Patients with COVID-19 infection who received metformin developed lower levels of interleukins [30] and other inflammatory bio-markers compared to non-users [31]. In addition, patients with type 2 diabetes are likely to develop upper respiratory diseases as well as their complications as presented in **Figure 4**; for example, chronic obstructive pulmonary diseases [32].

Long-term treatment with metformin among patients with type 2 diabetes was linked with a decreased ratio of neutrophil/lymphocyte, compared with sulfonylurea antidiabetic drugs [33]. In addition, metformin showed a protective effect among patients with type 2 diabetes regarding pneumonia-related hospitalizations and mortality rates [34].

In a clinical trial comparing metformin with placebo, the study revealed that metformin decreases the extent of pneumonia and also all pro-inflammatory cytokines among treated patients when compared with the placebo group [35]. The metformin protective effects against pulmonary infections have been hypothesized according to several mechanisms. In lung injury induced by hypoxia in animal models, metformin reduced the level of inflammatory mediators; for example, cytokines IL-6 and TNF-alpha [36]. Such traps, when overexpressed may result in exaggerated inflammatory responses with damaging effects [37].

6.2 Breast cancer

Insulin resistance could frequently contribute to the co-existence of type 2 diabetes, obesity, and cancer. This insulin resistance would result in abnormal cell growth via over-stimulation of the insulin/insulin-like growth factor pathway [38]. Other epidemiological studies showed that glycemic variability adds also some burden to cancer-related death in type 2 diabetes [39]. In the case of breast cancer, metformin exerted anticancer effects by changing the metabolic environment. This is achieved via reducing the levels of circulating insulin by improving insulin resistance related to phosphoinositide 3-kinases (PI3K) signaling [40]. Activating AMPK and liver kinase B1 (LKB1) with metformin via inhibition mTOR pathway in cancer cells. This would ultimately reduce protein synthesis and cell growth [41]. In addition, the signal transducer and activator of transcription 3 (STAT3) play a contributing role through the AMPK and LKB1 pathway which activated apoptosis in triple-negative breast cancer. Metformin had also been shown to shift the balance of sphingosine phosphate toward ceramides which will result in the inhibition of cell growth. Additional anticancer actions of metformin involved increased oxidation of fatty acids and reduced transcription factors expression implicated in cancer proliferation [40].

Metformin-induced programmed cell death of cancer cells in experimental studies with inhibition of vascularization of tumor cells through vascular endothelial growth factor A. In addition, metformin proved its ability to increase patients' responses to programmed death-ligand 1 (PD-L1) chemotherapy via decreasing glucose and consumption by tumor cells [37]. Metformin also helps to overcome the chemoresistance of endometrial cancer cells by changing the epigenetic signature of tumor cells [38]. Metformin showed the ability to reduce the incidence of cancers as shown in several observational studies [39, 40]. A cohort study on patients in the UK showed that metformin monotherapy was associated with a decreased cancer risk, compared with antidiabetic sulfonylureas.

Activating the JNK/p38 MAPK pathway via metformin was proved to be contributing mechanism by metformin to induce an apoptosis-mediated effect. This would lead to growth inhibition and induce the expression of DNA damage-inducible gene 153 (GADD153) [41]. Tseng et al. provided data proposing that metformin could reduce MAPK-mediated paclitaxel-induced expression of excision repair cross complementary 1 [42]. Human epidermal growth factor receptor-2 (HER2) is a member of the epidermal growth factor receptor family. HER2 is overexpressed in nearly 20–30% of breast cancers. In human breast cancer cells, AMPK-independent inhibition of mTOR was induced by metformin which suppressed HER2 oncoprotein overexpression [43]. In addition, combination therapy of metformin with trastuzumab, anti-HER2 monoclonal antibody, could eliminate cancer stem cell populations in HER2-positive breast carcinoma cells [44].

Cancer stem cells, or tumor-initiating cells, are a group of cancer cells that have unlimited ability to regenerate resulting in tumorigenesis [45]. Cancer stem cells are believed to be both chemoresistant [46, 47] and radioresistant [48, 49]. They may be responsible for cancer metastasis and relapse, which are the major obstacle to increasing the overall survival of cancer patients. In 2009, the inhibition of cancer stem cells by metformin was first proven clinically among breast cancer models [50]. Subsequently, metformin was used as a chemo-sensitizers in cancer xenografts to eradicate cancer stem cells in multiple cancer types [51]. Metformin was able to suppress cell proliferation and migration in pancreatic cancer by deregulating miRNAs of cancer stem cells [52]. In addition, metformin inhibits esophageal and made cells more sensitive cells to 5-fluorouracil cytotoxic effects leading to the inhibition of cancer cell growth [53]. Song et al. reported that the mechanism by which metformin targets cancer stem cells is via increasing the sensitivity to radiotherapy. This would activate AMPK and suppress mTOR and help to overcome radioresistance of cancer stem cells [54].

6.3 Degenerative and cognitive disorders

Type 2 diabetes frequently coexists with aging and cognitive dysfunction. Alzheimer's disease (AD) involves the formation of beta-amyloid plaques, neuroinflammation, and neuronal loss which causes dementia in patients with or without type 2 diabetes. Metformin demonstrated some capabilities in some experimental studies to prevent amyloid plaque formation via AMPK-dependent mechanisms [55]. Metformin improved neuro-glial cell differentiation and survival at the microenvironment level partially due to its anti-inflammatory effects [56]. Additionally, metformin might facilitate infarction-induced neural tissue repair which is done via favoring an M2 phenotype [57]. In animal studies, metformin-treated rats demonstrated a reversal of cognitive impairment caused by scopolamine [58]. In a rat model of forebrain ischemia, metformin treatment over 7 days in a rat model of forebrain ischemia resulted in the restoration of regulation of the AMPK-derived neurotrophic factor/protein S6 kinase mechanism with enhanced learning and memory [59]. One of the main confounders of the effects of metformin on cognitive function is its inhibitory effect on vitamin B12 intestinal absorption [60, 61]. In a pilot study including nondiabetic adults, a daily dose of 2 g metformin for a treatment time of 8 weeks was associated with improvement in executive function and other measures related to learning, attention capacity, and memory [62]. Taken together, these results suggested that metformin showed favorable effects on cognitive function depending on the duration and dose of metformin treatment.

7. Conclusions

In conclusion, metformin has been recognized and efficiently used in the treatment of several metabolic disorders, infectious, and inflammatory diseases [63]. Having an enzyme capable to catalyze several reactions (Promiscuous enzyme); for example, lipase enzyme which is capable to convert lipids or phospholipids or triglycerides to corresponding fatty acids and alcohols.

Moreover, having a drug with a unique chemical feature, multiple therapeutic targets, high safety therapeutic margin, and affordable economic cost [64, 65] may contribute to reducing mortality and improving recovery due to pandemic diseases; for example, COVID-19 and its fatal complications.

8. Future perspective

Nowadays, degenerative diseases, cancer, autism, psychological disorders, and many other genetic diseases may be targeted by the newly developed polyfunctional or mult-target drugs.

Recently, poly-targets molecules including metformin have been recognized and efficiently used in the treatment of several metabolic disorders, infectious, and inflammatory diseases. The capability of small molecules or drugs to react in a selective manner with different receptors to produce broad pharmacological effects may pose another useful class of promiscuity.

We do encourage all researchers to work vividly to develop as many multi-drugs as we can either via choosing a combination of different pharmacophores from single-target ligands or via the selection of preferentially expressed protein/antigen as manifested in many infectious diseases or cancer or via examining the possible ligand (drug) interact with a receptor (target) to figure out the existing energy and possible extent of interaction.

Acknowledgements

The authors would like to acknowledge the great help and support of STDF, for the continuous support and financial fund for STDF grant within the framework of the German Egyptian Research Fund (GERF), Project ID: 33601, "A novel innovative Approach for the Optimization of Phyto-pharmaceuticals: Modulation of Medicinal plants Constituents by Elicitation", Principal Investigator: Farid A. Badria. Also, the authors would like to acknowledge the contribution of Mr. Mohamed G. Farrag, Faculty of Pharmacy, Mansoura University, Mansoura 35516 Egypt for his valuable graphic work.

Conflict of interest

No conflict of interest.

Abbreviations

AD	Alzheimer's disease
AMPK	Adenosine monophosphate-activated protein kinase
CAD	Computer-assisted drug
cAMP	Cyclic adenosine monophosphate
CHDs	Complex health disorders
COVID-19	Coronavirus disease of 2019
CVS	Cardiovascular system
eNOS	Endothelial nitric oxide synthase also referred to as NOS3 or NOSIII
FDA	Food and Drugs Administration
GADD153	Growth arrest- and DNA damage-inducible gene 153
GIT	Gastrointestinal tract

Author details

Farid A. Badria[1*], Ahmed R. Ali[2], Ahmed Elbermawi[1], Yhiya Amen[1] and Adel F. Badria[3]

1 Faculty of Pharmacy, Department of Pharmacognosy, Mansoura University, Mansoura, Egypt

2 Medicinal Chemistry, Faculty of Pharmacy, Mansoura University, Mansoura, Egypt

3 Department of Fibre and Polymer Technology, KTH Royal Institute of Technology, Stockholm, Sweden

*Address all correspondence to: badri002@mans.edu.eg

References

[1] Badria FA, Ahmed MH. Multi-targets drugs: A new therapeutic approach. International Journal of Research in Pharmaceutical and Nano Sciences. 2018;7(5):205-213

[2] Badria FA. Drug Repurposing – Hypothesis, Molecular Aspects and Therapeutic Applications. London, UK, Rijeka: IntechOpen; 2020

[3] Koeberle A, Werz O. Multi-target approach for natural products in inflammation. Drug Discovery Today. 2014;**19**(12):1871-1882. DOI: 10.1016/j.drudis.2014.08.006

[4] Xie L, Xie L, Kinnings SL, Bourne PE. Novel computational approaches to polypharmacology as a means to define responses to individual drugs. Annual Review of Pharmacology and Toxicology. 2012;**52**(1):361-379. DOI: 10.1146/annurev-pharmtox-010611-134630

[5] Kell D. Finding novel pharmaceuticals in the systems biology era using multipleeffective drug targets, phenotypic screeningand knowledge of transporters: Where drugdiscovery went wrong and how to fix it. The FEBS Journal. 2013;**280**(23):5957-5980

[6] Talevi A. Multi-target pharmacology: Possibilities and limitations of the 'skeleton key approach' from a medicinal chemist perspective. Frontiers in Pharmacology. 22 Sep 2015;**6**:205. DOI: 10.3389/fphar.2015.00205. PMID: 26441661; PMCID: PMC4585027

[7] Zimmermann GR, Lehár J, Keith CT. Multi-target therapeutics: When the whole is greater than the sum of the parts. Drug Discovery Today. 2007;**12**(1-2):34-42. DOI: 10.1016/j.drudis.2006.11.008

[8] Ashburn TT, Thor KB. Drug repositioning: Identifying new uses for existing drugs. Nature Reviews. Drug Discovery. 2004;**3**(8):673-683

[9] Novac N. Challenges and opportunities of drug repositioning. Trends in Pharmacological Sciences. 2013;**34**(5):267-272

[10] Mori A. Guanidines: Historical, Biological, Biochemical, and Clinical Aspects of the Naturally Occurring Guanidine Compounds. London: Springer; 1985

[11] Mondal S, Samajdar RN, Mukherjee S, Bhattacharyya AJ, Bagchi B. Unique features of metformin: A combined experimental, theoretical, and simulation study of its structure, dynamics, and interaction energetics with DNA grooves. The Journal of Physical Chemistry. B. 2018;**122**(8):2227-2242. DOI: 10.1021/acs.jpcb.7b11928

[12] Sterne J. Pharmacology and mode of action of the hypoglycemic guanidine derivatives. In: Campbell GD, editor. Oral Hypoglycemic Agents. New York, USA: Academic Press; 1969. pp. 193-245

[13] Bailey CJ, Turner RC. Metformin. The New England Journal of Medicine. 1996;**334**(9):574-579. DOI: 10.1056/NEJM199602293340906

[14] Muller HRH. Pharmacology of galegin. Archiv fur Experimentelle Pathologie und Pharmakologie. 1927;**125**:212-228

[15] Lamoia TE, Shulman GI. Cellular and molecular mechanisms of metformin action. Endocrine Reviews. 2021;**42**:77-96

[16] Lv Z, Guo Y. Metformin and its benefits for various diseases. Frontiers in Endocrinology. 2020;**11**:191

[17] Gurung M et al. Role of gut microbiota in type 2 diabetes pathophysiology. eBioMedicine. 2020;**51**:102590. DOI: 10.1016/j.ebiom.2019.11.051

[18] Hsu S-K et al. New insight into the effects of metformin on diabetic retinopathy, aging and cancer: Nonapoptotic cell death, immunosuppression, and effects beyond the AMPK pathway. International Journal of Molecular Sciences. 2021;**22**(17):9453. DOI: 10.3390/ijms22179453

[19] Holman RR, Paul SK, Bethel MA, Matthews DR, Neil HAW. 10-year follow-up of intensive glucose control in type 2 diabetes. The New England Journal of Medicine. 2008;**359**(15):1577-1589. DOI: 10.1056/NEJMoa0806470

[20] Aroda VR et al. Metformin for diabetes prevention: Insights gained from the Diabetes Prevention Program/ Diabetes Prevention Program Outcomes Study. Diabetologia. 2017;**60**(9):1601-1611. DOI: 10.1007/s00125-017-4361-9

[21] de Jager J et al. Long-term effects of metformin on endothelial function in type 2 diabetes: A randomized controlled trial. Journal of Internal Medicine. 2014;**275**(1):59-70. DOI: 10.1111/joim.12128

[22] Triggle CR, Ding H. Metformin is not just an antihyperglycaemic drug but also has protective effects on the vascular endothelium. Acta Physiologica. 2017;**219**:138-151

[23] Marfella R et al. Metformin improves hemodynamic and rheological responses to L-arginine in NIDDM patients. Diabetes Care. 1996;**19**(9):934-939. DOI: 10.2337/diacare.19.9.934

[24] Grant PJ. Beneficial effects of metformin on haemostasis and vascular function in man. Diabetes & Metabolism. 2003;**29**:6-44

[25] Dalan R. Metformin, neutrophils and COVID-19 infection. Diabetes Research and Clinical Practice. 2020;**164**:108230

[26] Sharma S, Ray A, Sadasivam B. Metformin in COVID-19: A possible role beyond diabetes. Diabetes Research and Clinical Practice. 2020;**164**:108183. DOI: 10.1016/j.diabres.2020.108183

[27] Bramante CT et al. Metformin and risk of mortality in patients hospitalised with COVID-19: A retrospective cohort analysis. Lancet Healthy Longevity. 2021;**2**(1):e34-e41. DOI: 10.1016/S2666-7568(20)30033-7

[28] Poly TN, Islam MM, Li Y-C(J), Lin M-C, Hsu M-H, Wang Y-C. Metformin use is associated with decreased mortality in COVID-19 patients with diabetes: Evidence from retrospective studies and biological mechanism. Journal of Clinical Medicine. 2021;**10**(16):3507. DOI: 10.3390/jcm10163507

[29] Chen Y et al. Clinical characteristics and outcomes of patients with diabetes and COVID-19 in association with glucose-lowering medication. Diabetes Care. 2020;**43**(7):1399-1407. DOI: 10.2337/dc20-0660

[30] Cheng X et al. Metformin is associated with higher incidence of acidosis, but not mortality, in individuals with COVID-19 and pre-existing type 2 diabetes. Cell Metabolism. 2020;**32**(4):537-547.e3. DOI: 10.1016/j.cmet.2020.08.013

[31] de Jager CPC et al. The neutrophil-lymphocyte count ratio in patients with community-acquired pneumonia. PLoS One. 2012;7(10):e46561. DOI: 10.1371/journal.pone.0046561

[32] Cameron AR et al. Anti-inflammatory effects of metformin irrespective of diabetes status. Circulation Research. 2016;**119**(5):652-665. DOI: 10.1161/CIRCRESAHA.116.308445

[33] Mor A, Petersen I, Sørensen HT, Thomsen RW. Metformin and other glucose-lowering drug initiation and rates of community-based antibiotic use and hospital-treated infections in patients with type 2 diabetes: A Danish nationwide population-based cohort study. BMJ Open. 2016;**6**(8):e011523. DOI: 10.1136/bmjopen-2016-011523

[34] Pernicova I et al. Metformin to reduce metabolic complications and inflammation in patients on systemic glucocorticoid therapy: A randomised, double-blind, placebo-controlled, proof-of-concept, phase 2 trial. The Lancet Diabetes and Endocrinology. 2020;**8**(4):278-291. DOI: 10.1016/S2213-8587(20)30021-8

[35] Chen X et al. Metformin attenuates hyperoxia-induced lung injury in neonatal rats by reducing the inflammatory response. American Journal of Physiology-Lung Cellular and Molecular Physiology. 2015;**309**(3):L262-L270. DOI: 10.1152/ajplung.00389.2014

[36] Menegazzo L et al. The antidiabetic drug metformin blunts NETosis in vitro and reduces circulating NETosis biomarkers in vivo. Acta Diabetologica. 2018;**55**(6):593-601. DOI: 10.1007/s00592-018-1129-8

[37] Singhal A et al. Metformin as adjunct antituberculosis therapy. Science Translational Medicine. 2014;**6**(263, 263):159. DOI: 10.1126/scitranslmed.3009885

[38] Yang X, Lee HM, Chan JCN. Drug–subphenotype interactions for cancer in type 2 diabetes mellitus. Nature Reviews. Endocrinology. 2015;**11**(6):372-379. DOI: 10.1038/nrendo.2015.37

[39] Mao D et al. Risk associations of long-term HbA1c variability and obesity on cancer events and cancer-specific death in 15,286 patients with diabetes - A prospective cohort study. Lancet Regional Health – Western Pacific. 2022;**18**:100315. DOI: 10.1016/j.lanwpc.2021.100315

[40] Vancura A, Bu P, Bhagwat M, Zeng J, Vancurova I. Metformin as an anticancer agent. Trends in Pharmacological Sciences. 2018;**39**(10):867-878. DOI: 10.1016/j.tips.2018.07.006

[41] Heckman-Stoddard BM, DeCensi A, Sahasrabuddhe VV, Ford LG. Repurposing metformin for the prevention of cancer and cancer recurrence. Diabetologia. 2017;**60**(9):1639-1647. DOI: 10.1007/s00125-017-4372-6

[42] Scharping NE, Menk AV, Whetstone RD, Zeng X, Delgoffe GM. Efficacy of PD-1 blockade is potentiated by metformin-induced reduction of tumor hypoxia. Cancer Immunology Research. 2017;**5**(1):9-16. DOI: 10.1158/2326-6066.CIR-16-0103

[43] Bai M et al. Metformin sensitizes endometrial cancer cells to chemotherapy through IDH1-induced Nrf2 expression via an epigenetic mechanism. Oncogene. 2018;**37**(42):5666-5681. DOI: 10.1038/s41388-018-0360-7

[44] Mallik R, Chowdhury TA. Metformin in cancer. Diabetes Research and Clinical Practice. 2018;**143**:409-419

[45] Bodmer M, Meier C, Krähenbühl S, Jick SS, Meier CR. Long-term metformin use is associated with decreased risk of breast cancer. Diabetes Care.

2010;**33**(6):1304-1308. DOI: 10.2337/dc09-1791

[46] Wu N, Gu C, Gu H, Hu H, Han Y, Li Q. "Metformin induces apoptosis of lung cancer cells through activating JNK/p38 MAPK pathway and GADD153." Neoplasma. 2011;58(6):482-490. DOI: 10.4149/neo_2011_06_482

[47] Tseng S-C et al. Metformin-mediated downregulation of p38 mitogen-activated protein kinase-dependent excision repair cross-complementing 1 decreases DNA repair capacity and sensitizes human lung cancer cells to paclitaxel. Biochemical Pharmacology. 2013;**85**(4):583-594. DOI: 10.1016/j.bcp.2012.12.001

[48] Vazquez-Martin A, Oliveras-Ferraros C, Menendez JA. The antidiabetic drug metformin suppresses HER2 (erbB-2) oncoprotein overexpression via inhibition of the mTOR effector p70S6K1 in human breast carcinoma cells. Cell Cycle. 2009;**8**(1):88-96. DOI: 10.4161/cc.8.1.7499

[49] Vazquez-Martin A, Oliveras-Ferraros C, Del Barco S, Martin-Castillo B, Menendez JA. The anti-diabetic drug metformin suppresses self-renewal and proliferation of trastuzumab-resistant tumor-initiating breast cancer stem cells. Breast Cancer Research and Treatment. 2011;**126**(2):355-364. DOI: 10.1007/s10549-010-0924-x

[50] Reya T, Morrison SJ, Clarke MF, Weissman IL. Stem cells, cancer, and cancer stem cells. Nature. 2001;**414**(6859):105-111. DOI: 10.1038/35102167

[51] Dalerba P, Cho RW, Clarke MF. Cancer stem cells: Models and concepts. Annual Review of Medicine. 2007;**58**(1):267-284. DOI: 10.1146/annurev.med.58.062105.204854

[52] Ma S, Lee TK, Zheng B-J, Chan KW, Guan X-Y. CD133+ HCC cancer stem cells confer chemoresistance by preferential expression of the Akt/PKB survival pathway. Oncogene. 2008;**27**(12):1749-1758. DOI: 10.1038/sj.onc.1210811

[53] Bao S et al. Glioma stem cells promote radioresistance by preferential activation of the DNA damage response. Nature. 2006;**444**(7120):756-760. DOI: 10.1038/nature05236

[54] Phillips TM, WH MB, Pajonk F. The response of CD24(-/low)/CD44+ breast cancer-initiating cells to radiation. Journal of the National Cancer Institute. 2006;**98**:1777-1785

[55] Ou Z et al. Metformin treatment prevents amyloid plaque deposition and memory impairment in APP/PS1 mice. Brain, Behavior, and Immunity. 2018;**69**:351-363. DOI: 10.1016/j.bbi.2017.12.009

[56] Hardie DG. AMP-activated protein kinase: Maintaining energy homeostasis at the cellular and whole-body levels. Annual Review of Nutrition. 2014;**34**:31-55

[57] Jin Q et al. Improvement of functional recovery by chronic metformin treatment is associated with enhanced alternative activation of microglia/macrophages and increased angiogenesis and neurogenesis following experimental stroke. Brain, Behavior, and Immunity. 2014;**40**:131-142. DOI: 10.1016/j.bbi.2014.03.003

[58] Mostafa DK, Ismail CA, Ghareeb DA. Differential metformin dose-dependent effects on cognition in rats: Role of Akt. Psychopharmacologia. 2016;**233**:2513-2524

[59] Ghadernezhad N, Khalaj L, Pazoki-Toroudi H, Mirmasoumi M,

Ashabi G. Metformin pretreatment enhanced learning and memory in cerebral forebrain ischaemia: The role of the AMPK/BDNF/P70SK signalling pathway. Pharmaceutical Biology. 2016;**54**(10):2211-2219. DOI: 10.3109/13880209.2016.1150306

[60] Moore E, Mander A, Ames D, Carne R, Sanders K, Watters D. Cognitive impairment and vitamin B12: A review. International Psychogeriatrics. 2012;**24**(4):541-556. DOI: 10.1017/S1041610211002511

[61] Moore EM et al. Increased risk of cognitive impairment in patients with diabetes is associated with metformin. Diabetes Care. 2013;**36**(10):2981-2987. DOI: 10.2337/dc13-0229

[62] Koenig AM et al. Effects of the insulin sensitizer metformin in alzheimer disease. Alzheimer Disease and Associated Disorders. 2017;**31**(2):107-113. DOI: 10.1097/WAD.0000000000000202

[63] Atici Y, Baskol G, Bayram F. A new approach for the pleiotropic effect of metformin use in type 2 diabetes mellitus. Turkish Journal of Biochemistry. 2 May 2022:1-6. DOI: 10.1515/tjb-2022-0013

[64] Wu H et al. Metformin: A promising drug for human cancers (Review). Oncology Letters. 2022;**24**(1):204. DOI: 10.3892/ol.2022.13325

[65] Abdool Karim SS, Devnarain N. Time to stop using ineffective COVID-19 drugs. The New England Journal of Medicine. 2022;**387**(7): 654-655. DOI: 10.1056/NEJMe2209017

Section 2

Update in Metformin and Diabetes

Chapter 2

Pharmacogenetics of Metformin in Type 2 Diabetes: Perspectives for Latin America

Eloy A. Zepeda-Carrillo, Rafael Torres Valadez, Sara A. Campos Huerta and Elisa María Barrón Cabrera

Abstract

Metformin, in the anti-hyperglycemic pharmacological therapy, is consumed by more than 150 million people annually in the world due to its affordable price, safety, and because of considerable pleiotropic effect that has a positive impact on the control of glycemia, insulin resistance, cardiovascular health, and cancer in patients with type 2 diabetes (T2D). Differences in metformin's effect on glycemic control have been associated with diet, abdominal obesity, years of T2D evolutions, and genetic factors. The Population of Latin America presents an important genetic component of Amerindians that could be explained to some extent in the response to metformin in glycemic control. The most recognized effect of metformin is to inhibit gluconeogenesis hepatica. In recent years, it has been observed to reduce the effect on body mass, positive effects on inflammation, and recently on the intestine with changes in the microbiome that favor suppression of postprandial hyperglycemia. Association studies between genetic variants coding for proteins related to metformin pharmacodynamics have shown different effects on glycemic control in several ethnic groups with European and Asian ancestry, but in Latin America they are scarce or none. Nutrients can interact with metformin favoring or decreasing its anti-hyperglycemic effect, so the diet should be considered.

Keywords: metformin, type 2 diabetes, genes, pharmacogenetics, nutrigenetics, Latin America

1. Introduction

Type 2 diabetes (TD2) shows an upward trend in its prevalence globally, and in the developing countries of Latin America, an increase of up to 50% is estimated by 2045 [1, 2]. Drug treatment to control hyperglycemia in these patients is a daily challenge at the first level of medical care. Metformin is a biguanide that is prescribed as the first drug of choice to control blood glucose based on the treatment guidelines issued by the European Association for the Study of Diabetes (EASD) and the American Association for the Study of Diabetes (ADA), due to its efficacy and safety as well as its low cost which makes this drug widely accessible in any socioeconomic stratum [3]. The main effect shown by this biguanide is the suppression of hepatic glucose production, but the complete mechanism is not fully demonstrated. Despite the anti-hyperglycemic therapeutic effects demonstrated in several trials since the 1950s of the last century, no more than 35% of patients with this pharmacotherapy achieve the expected glycemic control. In addition, the gastrointestinal side effects of this drug are a reason for non-adherence to treatment, which explains why many patients seek alternatives and delay their therapeutic goal. To explain these effects of metformin, studies have been carried out focused on pharmacokinetics and pharmacodynamics that have shown the important role of proteins related to its intestinal absorption as well as its uptake hepatic. The organic cation transporters OCT1, OCT2, and OCT3 have gained relevance to understanding to a large extent the effects described by metformin to date [4].

Studies of gene variants that code for these proteins and their association with the anti-hyperglycemic effect of metformin in subjects with TD2, have shown that the genetic component of the patient is decisive to explain the anti-hyperglycemic effect of this drug, as well as its gastrointestinal side effects. The focus of these gene-drug association studies has been achieved thanks to the development of Pharmacogenetics [5]. The first pharmacogenetic studies in TD2 emerged in Europe and Asia, and later in the United States of America. From genome-wide association studies (GWAS) in some cohorts, genes with the statistical association of response to metformin were found which are not directly related to the action of the drug, so its usefulness was not expected. Thanks to metformin pharmacodynamic studies it was possible to conduct association studies with candidate genes such as those encoding the organic cation transporters OCT1, OCT2, and OCT3, mainly. The solute carrier family 22 (SLC22) genes encode for these transporters of organic cations located in the plasmatic membranes of intestinal, hepatic, and renal cells, where metformin has its absorption, anti-hyperglycemic effect, and excretion, respectively [5]. The SLC22A1/OCT1 gene encodes for the OCT1 transporter and has been the most explored for its close relationship with the effect of metformin on the liver. More than 30 polymorphic variants of this gene have been described and their association with the effect of metformin has been variable in different populations with TD2. Among the most studied SLC22A1/OCT1 gene polymorphisms in recent times is *Met*408*Val* rs628031, whose frequency of the risk allele variant A (408*Val*) reported for America in the 1000 Genome Project Phase 3 is the lowest [6, 7].

Diet is another factor that affects glycemic control and the therapeutic response of metformin in patients with TD2. The diet of Latin American countries has been modified in recent years influenced by the Westernized diet that is high in saturated fats, simple sugars, cholesterol, and low in fiber which has an impact on the elevation of blood glucose that impacts the expected anti-hyperglycemic effect of metformin. Therapeutic dietary approaches to contribute to glycemic control in TD2 have focused on caloric balance and the percentage contribution of macronutrients in the total color intake of the patient's requirement. The studies of the association of genes with specific nutrients in the diet have begun to demonstrate the importance of the genetic component in response to specific macro or micronutrients, which has allowed the development of nutrigenetics.

2. Epidemiology impact of T2D and their comorbidities in Latin America

The prevalence of diabetes in Latin America in adults in 2019 ranged from less than 6% in Ecuador and Argentina to 17% in Belize. On average, the prevalence for Latin

America was 9.7%, with an increase of 7.4% compared to 2010. The largest increase was 10 percentage points recorded in Belize, while the largest decrease was 6 percentage points recorded in Uruguay and Venezuela between 2010 and 2019 [1]. Other countries where it decreased were Peru, Panama, and Ecuador but with less than 5 percentage points in the same period. Two Latin American countries that are Brazil and Mexico in the global Top Ten of T2D with sixth and seventh place, respectively, contributing almost 30 million people with diabetes in general globally [8]. When considering the Americas region, the World Health Organization WHO includes Canada and the USA. In the Region of America, about 62 million people have T2D, contributing 15% to the global prevalence of 422 million individuals diagnosed with T2D that was reported in 2014, and with a trend towards an increase in cases. In the Americas region, prevalence has tripled since 1980 and is estimated to reach 109 million by 2040 [2]. In 2019, diabetes was the sixth leading cause of death, with an estimated 244,084 deaths directly caused by T2D. In addition, it is the second leading cause of disability-adjusted life years (DALY's), which reflects the limiting complications for their daily activity that people with T2D suffer throughout their lives. In North America and the Caribbean alone, 1 in 7 adults lives with T2D (51 million) and is expected to reach 57 million adults by 2030 and 63 million by 2045. In this region, it caused 931,000 deaths and 415 million USD was spent due to this disease in the year 2021 alone [9, 10].

The International Diabetes Federation (IDF) divides the Americas region into North America and the Caribbean (NAC), and South and Central America (SACA). The NAC region has the second highest prevalence of diabetes among IDF regions at 14% and the number of people with diabetes for this region is projected to increase by 24% to 63 million by 2045. Of this region, Mexico is the second with the largest population with diabetes (14.1 million), below the USA. In this NAC region, mortality from diabetes is the second highest with 931,000 and the second highest percentage with 18.4%, in people of working age. In the SACA region, it is estimated that 1 day in 11 adults has diabetes (about 33 million), and it is estimated that it will increase by 50%, that is, to 49 million in 2045. Of this region (SACA), Brazil is in first place with the highest number of people with diabetes (15.7 million), followed by Colombia (3.4 million), Venezuela (2.3 million), Argentina (8 million), and Chile (1.7 million [9]. In the NACA region, 415 billion USD was spent due to this disease, while the SACA region 65 billion USD was spent [9]. In addition, Brazil of the SACA region and Mexico of the NAC, are two Latin American countries that are in third and eighth place with the highest total expenditure due to diabetes with 42.9 and 19.9 USD billion, respectively, [9]. Of these amounts reported by the IFD in its Diabetes Atlas, about 90% of the total of these amounts correspond to TD2.

Projections on the prevalence of TD2 estimate that developing countries will be among those with the greatest increase due to the social determinants of health such as diet, physical activity, access to health systems for timely diagnosis, and the budget available for TD2 care. The increase in population in urban areas and the consequent "Westernized" type diet in combination with a decrease in physical activity favor overweight and obesity which are risk factors for the development of TD2, which allow us to assume an unfavorable future for the control of TD2 and its comorbidities in this geographical region.

2.1 Pharmacotherapy with metformin in TD2

In medieval times, the plant *Galega officinalis* (Galega or French lilac) was used in Europe as a popular remedy to treat diabetes. Phytochemical studies in the late 1800s revealed that the plant was rich in guanidine. In 1918, animal studies showed that guanidine had hypoglycemic effects, but with toxic effects for clinical use. In 1929 the biguanide "metformin" was synthesized, which demonstrated the hypoglycemic effects observed by biguanide, but without the toxic effects [4]. The first clinical trial using metformin to treat T2D was reported in 1957. In the mid-1950s of the last century, metformin was approved in Europe as a treatment for T2D and in the United States of America (USA) since1995 [4]. After more than 60 years of clinical use for T2D, metformin has demonstrated safety and efficacy, making it the most commonly prescribed oral drug globally to control T2D [4]. Metformin is prescribed as the first choice of anti-hyperglycemic treatment worldwide, based on international guidelines for the management of T2D issued by the European Association for the Study of Diabetes (EASD) and the American Diabetes Association (ADA) [3]. Metformin is taken by about 150 million people each year for its safety, efficacy, and low cost, in addition to the pleiotropic effects that have a positive impact on glycemic control, insulin resistance, cardiovascular health, and cancer in patients with T2D [11]. In addition, metformin improves the inflammatory effects associated with obesity and reduces body mass, which is why it is widely prescribed in Mexico and the USA, where the prevalence of overweight and obesity is high [12, 13]. Despite the beneficial effects described, only about 30% achieve the goal of glycemic control (HbA1c <7%), so the pharmacokinetics and pharmacodynamics of this drug have been studied to explain these results. Studies in this regard have shown that in the intestine, the Organic Cation Transporter (OCT1 and OCT3), a protein with transmembrane channel functions in "enterocyte" epithelial cell, is responsible for the absorption of metformin, while in the liver this same protein is responsible for internalizing it to exert one of the main anti-hyperglycemic effects, suppression of hepatic glucose production "hepatic gluconeogenesis," and in the kidney OCT1 and OCT2 are the route of excretion of metformin (**Figure 1**). This knowledge has allowed the search for genetic variants in the SLC22A1/OCT1 gene which codes for the OCT1 protein, associated with response to metformin with a disciplined approach known as Pharmacogenetics.

2.2 Mechanism of action of metformin and its effect on T2D

Although it is recognized that the main effect of metformin is the suppression of hepatic glucose production, this drug has multiple mechanisms of action and the clear benefits of its use in the treatment of T2D in relation to glucose metabolism are complex and not fully understood [14]. Physiologically, metformin has been shown to have a key role in the liver and intestine. At the molecular level, evidence shows that metformin acts by mechanisms related to AMP-activated protein kinase (AMPK) and by inhibition of mitochondrial respiration, which improves blood glucose by acting on these mechanisms, both dependent and independent mechanisms [15].

Traditionally, metformin acts on the liver through organic cation transporters 1 (OCT1), which absorbs the drug from the enterocytes into the portal vein through the basolateral membrane and enters the hepatocyte, reducing hepatic glucose production after a high-fat diet, which improves blood glucose levels [16]. In this context, metformin reduces hepatic gluconeogenesis by inhibiting respiratory chain complex I, which suppresses ATP production and increases cytoplasmic AMP → ATP and ADP → ATP ratios, changes that activate AMPK mechanisms, which is the main cellular bioenergetic sensor (**Figure 2**). Due to membrane potentials, metformin accumulates up to 1000 times more within the mitochondria than in the cytoplasm of

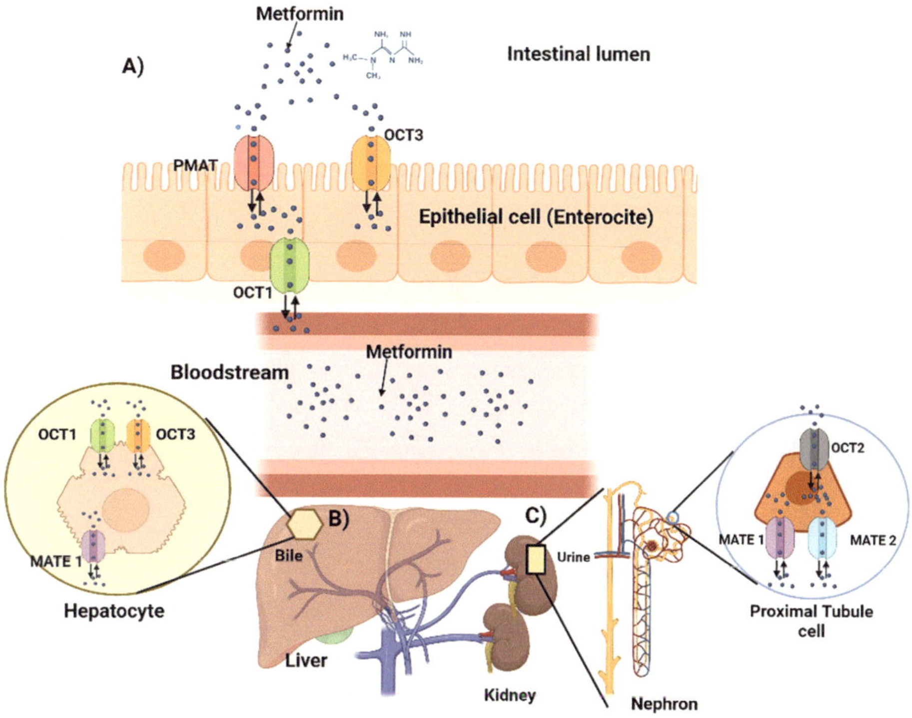

Figure 1.
Metformin pharmacodynamics. Scheme with the transporters responsible for the absorption, distribution, and elimination of metformin. (A) Intestinal absorption through the plasma membrane monoamine transporter (PMAT) and the Organic Cation Transporter 3 (OCT3), once in the "enterocyte" epithelial cell the Organic Cation Transporter 1 (OCT1) which is located on the basolateral surface, transports metformin to the serosal side of the endothelium, allowing its arrival in the bloodstream; (B) the transporters OCT1 and OCT3 are expressed in the sinusoidal membrane of hepatocytes where they capture metformin from the bloodstream. The elimination of metformin from inside the hepatocyte is by the Toxic Compound and Multidrug Extrusion Transporter (MATE1) helping to excrete metformin in bile, although in humans most of the metformin is excreted in the urine through MATE1; (C) the uptake of metformin from the bloodstream to renal epithelial cells is mainly facilitated by the Organic Cation Transporter 2 (OCT2) located on the basolateral membrane of renal proximal tubule cells, in turn, MATE1 and MATE2 expressed in the apical membrane of renal proximal tubule cells contribute to the excretion of metformin in the urine.

the cell, this energy-intensive process does not have the required supply of ATP and the concomitant suppression of this pathway could explain the effects obtained in the T2D treatment [17].

The effect of metformin on hepatic gluconeogenesis goes beyond mitochondrial control. Increases in the AMP → ATP ratio directly affect the activity of fructose-1,6-bisphosphatase, one of the key enzymes in this metabolic pathway, resulting in its acute inhibition. Due to the cellular energy imbalance, AMPK seeks to restore energy homeostasis by activating the catabolic pathways that generate ATP while deactivating the cellular processes that consume ATP. Activated AMPK phosphorylates the ACC1 and ACC2 isoforms of acetyl-CoA carboxylase (ACC), which inhibits fat synthesis and promotes fat oxidation, reducing hepatic lipid stores and improving hepatic insulin sensitivity in T2D patients [18, 19].

Although AMPK activation has not yet been determined exactly how it occurs, in this sense the effect of metformin is extremely complex and occurs at multiple levels by phosphorylating binding proteins, disassembling transcriptional coactivation complexes, and even deacetylating proteins that limit the rate of energy

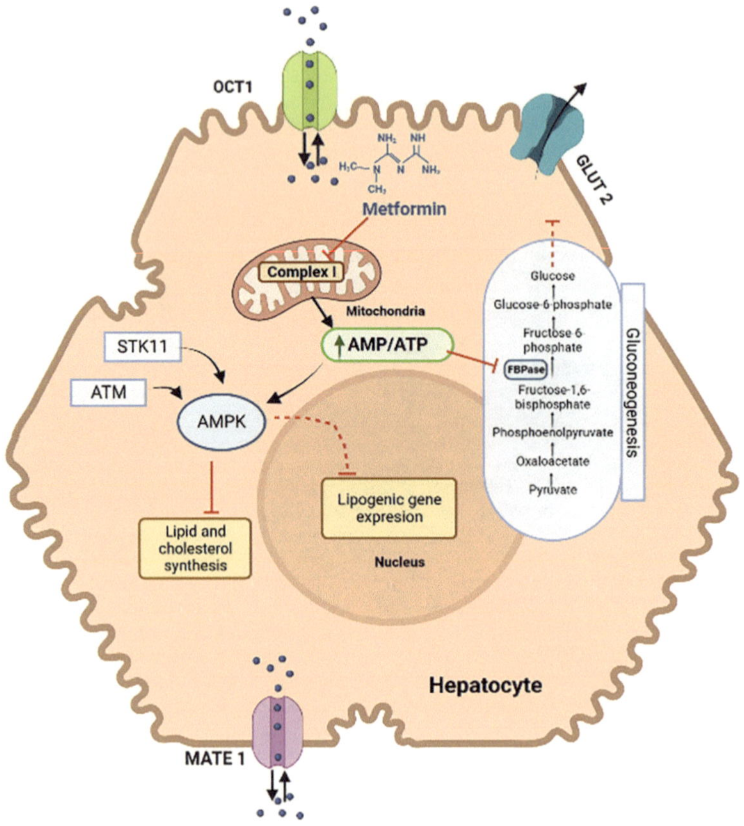

Figure 2.
Mechanism of action of metformin in the liver. Metformin reduces hepatic gluconeogenesis by inhibiting respiratory chain complex I, which suppresses ATP production and increases cytoplasmic AMP/ATP. Increases in the AMP/ATP ratio directly affect the activity of fructose-1,6-bisphosphatase, one of the key enzymes in gluconeogenesis, resulting in its acute inhibition. In addition, those changes activate AMP-activated protein kinase (AMPK), which is the main cellular bioenergetic sensor. Activation of AMPK results in the inhibition of lipogenic gene expression and cholesterol synthesis. AMPK activity may also be modulated by metformin through kinases such as the serine/threonine kinase encoded by ataxia telangiectasia mutated gene (ATM) or serine/threonine kinase 11 (STK11). FBPase, fructose-1,6-biphosphatase; GLUT 2, glucose transporter; MATE, Toxic Compound and Multidrug Extrusion Transporter.

biosynthesis [20]. Even if controversies persist about the effects of metformin on AMPK, the reduction in the expression of mRNAs encoding key enzymes of hepatic gluconeogenesis, and the improvement in hepatic insulin sensitivity, are proven long-term clinically relevant effects of metformin that are mediated by AMPK [21].

It has recently been postulated that the liver may not be the main target organ for metformin action in T2D patients as might be assumed. In this sense, in the gut, significant effects of metformin on anaerobic glucose metabolism have been observed. The reduction in net glucose uptake and the increase in lactate have made the intestines an important therapeutic target in the treatment of T2D with metformin, highlighting three main lines:

- Extended-release metformin is primarily retained in the gut, with minimal systemic absorption, and is as effective in lowering blood glucose as the standard formulation commonly implemented in T2D patients [22].

- The reduction of endogenous glucose production in the liver can only be partially explained by the effect of metformin, indicating the existence of other extrahepatic glucose-lowering mechanisms [23].

- Human studies have established that loss-of-function variants of the *SLC22A1* gene, encoding the OCT1 protein, reduce hepatic uptake of metformin but do not affect its efficacy in lowering HbA1c in T2D patients [24].

Metformin increases intestinal uptake of fluorodeoxyglucose in the colon, an effect that is accompanied by an increase in AMPK phosphorylation in colonic enterocytes, which affects energy homeostasis and glucose metabolism. In addition, at the intestinal level, metformin also affects glucose metabolism by increasing the secretion of glucagon-like peptide 1 (GLP-1), a mechanism of action that has been described for both immediate-release and prolonged-release metformin [25]. However, the potential mechanism of action of metformin mediated by the intestine that has recently generated the most interest has to do with the alteration of the intestinal microbiome and its inflammation.

In type 2 diabetes, metformin has been shown to have positive effects on intestinal inflammation, by inhibiting NF-κB signaling and differentiation of monocytes into macrophages, as well as suppression of proinflammatory cytokines from these macrophages [26]. In humans, metformin-dependent effects on the increase in *Escherichia spp.* and decrease in *Intestinibacter spp.* in the intestinal microbiome, have been linked to a decrease in adipose tissue inflammation and significant suppression of postprandial hyperglycemia [27]. This emphasizes that the changes in the microbiome in T2D are predominantly associated with the mechanism of action of metformin and not with the disease itself, although its role as a cause or consequence of the therapeutic effect still requires further investigation.

2.3 Pharmacogenetics of metformin in Latin America

From the development of technology with which it was possible to sequence the human genome and the software designs for the analysis of complete genomes that have emerged in the last decade, which are more accessible to the international scientific community, GWAS whole genome association studies have been generated to expand the knowledge of genes associated with susceptibility to develop T2D. Thus, since the first study of GWAS in T2D more than 100 loci of susceptibility have been described in different regions of the world. With the development of drugs for the treatment of hyperglycemia in TD2 with different effects and target tissues, studies have been carried out to advance the understanding of the variability in the response to these drugs based on the genetic component of the subjects studied. With this approach to determine the interindividual genetic variability of response to specific drugs arises pharmacogenetics, which focuses on the search for specific variants of genes whose expression products "proteins" are associated with lower pharmacological response (efficacy) or side effects to prescribed drugs.

The mechanisms of action of metformin have not been fully elucidated. Pharmacokinetic studies of metformin have shown that this biguanide is not metabolized in the body and is excreted without changes in its chemical composition through active tubular secretion in the urine by the kidney. With advances in the pharmacodynamics and pharmacokinetics of metformin, it has been possible to conduct studies in TD2 pharmacogenetics in several population groups in recent years. Until the end of 2020, about 30 genes have been found with specific variants associated with therapeutic response to metformin or side effects that limit their therapeutic use, so they are considered candidate genes. There are three large-scale genome-wide association studies (GWAS) conducted in different cohorts. In 2011, the first in a European cohort "Genetics of Diabetes Audit and Research Tayside" (GoDART) was completed and included 1024 patients affected by TD2 [28]. The main results of this study showed 14 single nucleotide polymorphisms (SNPs) mapped on chromosome 11 locus 11q22, which were successfully associated with treatment for achieving HbA1c $< 7\%$ goal in the 18 months after starting metformin treatment. Subsequently, the rs11212617 was studied in 2 independent cohorts, GoDARTS with 1783 patients treated with metformin and the UK Prospective Diabetes Cohort (UKPDS) with 1113 patients, resulting in a significant association with response to metformin in both studies [29]. This genetic variant rs11212617, is located in a large block of linkage disequilibrium, which includes a set of genes among which is the ATM gene, which had been one of the candidate genes in greater perspective since that study, by the replication of result emerged in other independent cohorts such as China Han and Western Saudi Arabia. However, no significant difference was found between the response to metformin and rs11212617 in patients with TD2 in the Iranian and Indian populations [5, 30]. The ATM gene encodes for a protein belonging to the PI3/PI4 kinase family whose function is an important cell cycle checkpoint, which is not directly related to pharmacodynamics, pharmacokinetics or described mechanisms of intracellular action of metformin [31].

In 2016, the Metformin Genetics (MetGen) Consortium conducted a three-stage GWAS that included nearly 13,500 participants from different ancestry. The SLC2A2 gene encoding the glucose transporter GLUT2, an integral membrane glycoprotein expressed in the intestine, liver, islet beta cells, and kidney, presented a C-allele variant rs8192675 with 0.17% ($p = 6.6 \times 10^{-14}$) greater metformin-induced HbA1c in 10,577 participants with European ancestry [32]. The association of this SNP rs8192675 with metformin response was replicated in the Germany Diabetes Study. In a meta-analysis with 13,123 participants of any ancestry (European, Latino, African American) the frequency of the C-allele associated with response to metformin varied widely, but there was no genetic heterogeneity between the different ethnic groups [32, 33].

The other GWAS-focused study that sought the association of genetic variants with HbA1c change in response to metformin pharmacotherapy in a TD2 cohort was the one applied in the cohort of Action to Control Cardiovascular Risk in Diabetes (ACCORD), which includes subjects from the USA. The rs254271 variant in PRPF31 gene and the variant rs2162145 in CYPA6 gene was found to be associated with worse and better responses to metformin, respectively ($p = 3.79 \times 10^{-6}$, beta $= 0.16$; $p = 4.04 \times 10^{-6}$, beta $= -0.197$), these results were similar in a meta-analysis of independent cohorts with response to metformin [34]. Previous studies that had identified the rs11212617 variant in the ATM gene and the rs8192675 variant in the SLC2A2 gene were not replicated in this study.

GWAS studies are very useful to identify genomic variants statistically associated with a given phenotype such as a disease. These early genetic association studies focused on the analysis of family-based linkage as well as candidate genes in small groups of TD2 patients. It has been observed that this approach to studies is usually useful only for the identification of genetic variants with large effects. Thus, the selection of candidate genes for the study of metformin response in patients with TD2 was then focused on genes coding for proteins related to the pharmacodynamics of this biguanide. Therefore, genes whose expression products such as organic cation transporters OCT are determinants for intestinal absorption, uptake liver, and renal excretion have been the most explored.

2.4 Pharmacogenetics of response to metformin in TD2 based on its pharmacodynamics

Organic cation transporters (OCT1, OCT2, and OCT3) are directly related to metformin pharmacodynamics as shown in **Figure 1**. The SLC22A1, SLC22A2, and SLC22A3 genes code for these proteins OCT1, OCT2, and OCT3. The OCT2 and OCT3 proteins are associated with intestinal absorption and renal clearance of metformin, so the genes that code for them have been studied more with side effects than with anti-hyperglycemic effects mainly. The OCT1 transporter is expressed in the intestine allowing its absorption, in the liver, it is the one that allows the entry to the hepatocyte to exert the anti-hyperglycemic effect by reducing hepatic gluconeogenesis and in the kidney for its elimination, which has become relevant for its close relationship with the efficacy of metformin [35, 36]. In humans, the SLC22A1/OCT1 gene (ID6580), located on the chromosome 6 locus (6q25.3), is among the most studied regarding the pharmacological response to metformin in glycemic control of patients with T2D. More than 30 polymorphic variants of this gene associated with different effects on metformin response have been identified in various ethnic groups, mostly from European and Asian regions, suggesting a population-specific response. At the end of the last decade, a systematic review highlighted and summarized the overall effects of polymorphisms in the SLC22A1/OCT1 gene in response to metformin and evaluated the role of these in interethnic differences. In total, 34 polymorphisms were found in 10 different ethnic groups. The response to metformin from these studies was measured with different variables such as %HbA1c, fasting plasma glucose (FPG), and postprandial plasma glucose (PPG). The *Met*408*Val* polymorphism of the SLC22A1/OCT1 gene (rs628031) has been the most widely studied with response to metformin and its genetic effect resulting in differences in glycemic control and side effects in the groups studied. This allows us to suggest the variable response of metformin based on the genetic variants according to the population studied [29]. These gene-metformin association studies have arisen in subjects with TD2 but with European and Asian ancestry mainly, which forces studies to be carried out in populations of Latin America, which presents a heterogeneity of ethnic groups with varied ancestry.

2.5 Global distribution of most studied SLC22A1/OCT1 gene variants with metformin response

The *Met*408*Val* polymorphism of the SLC22A1/OCT1 rs628031 gene has three A/C/G alleles, the ancestral allele G (Met 408) and the minor allele A (408Val), the latter associated with lower response to metformin. The global frequency reported in the 1000 Genomes Project Phase 3 for this SNP is 69% for the G allele and 31% for the A allele. The 1000 Genomes Project has the global regions defined in a particular way in Africa, America, East Asia, Europe, and Southeast Asia. For the Region of America, the frequency reported for the G allele is 78% and for the A allele 22%, whose frequency of the risk A allele is the lowest. While in Europe the frequency of allele G is 59% and for allele A is 41%, region that has the highest frequency of allele A. In the Southeast Asia region, the frequency is 61% for the G allele and 39% for the risk A allele, while in the African region the frequency of the G allele is 73% and 27% for the risk A allele [7]. With the frequency of the risk A allele in America at a low percentage compared to the other regions, a higher proportion of subjects with T2D who present a response to metformin for glycemic control would be expected. If we consider that Mexico and Brazil are two countries with a considerable prevalence of overweight and obesity in addition to TD2, which condition the metabolic control of these patients, metformin should be a promising drug to contribute to metabolic control in these subjects, but studies are required to determine the response to metformin considering in addition to these variant other variables of importance in TD2 such as age, years with TD2, physical activity, diet, among others. With these pharmacogenetic studies that are increasingly accessible, it is possible to demonstrate the association and magnitude of the effect of metformin in glycemic control that allows us to know who are the patients with TD2 responders of the non-responders to metformin, which will be a significant advance for the health of patients with TD2.

The SNP in gene SLC22A1/OCT1 rs594709 is another polymorphism that presents two variants, the ancestral allele A and the minor allele G, the latter associated with a lower response to metformin in glycemic control. The global frequency reported in the 1000 Genomes Project Phase 3 for this SNP is 68% for the G allele and 32% for the A allele. For the region of America, the frequency reported for allele A is 78% and 22% and for the risk allele G, the lowest frequency reported in all regions. While in Europe the frequency of allele A is 59% and 41% for allele G, a region that has the highest frequency of the risk allele G. The Southeast Asia region is the most frequent follower of the G risk allele with 39% and 61% for the A allele. In the African region, it has a frequency of 29% for the risk allele G and 71% for the allele A [37].

These two SNPs rs628031 and rs594709 show that their frequency in Latin America is the lowest compared to the other regions, as well as other SNPs studied in Europe and Asia. A la fecha se han encontrado cerca de 15 variantes geneticas asociadas con respuesta a metformina **Table 1**. In Latin America, the association studies of these SNPs should be an important issue to determine their association and magnitude with respect to the effect on glycemic control in different populations to approach the personalized medicine required by the patient with TD2. This personalized medicine would allow us to approach finding responders versus non-responders to establish metformin treatments with more patient achieving the therapeutic goal (%HbA1c <7).

2.6 Nutrition and dietary interactions between macro and micronutrients with metformin in T2D

Lifestyle modifications involve the incorporation of regular physical exercise, as well as complete, varied, sufficient, and balanced nutrition to ensure a correct supply of carbohydrates, protein, fiber, and polyunsaturated fats in patients with TD2, who present impaired metabolism of carbohydrates, lipids, and proteins. The typical nutritional approach includes a diet with caloric reduction to achieve weight loss and control the percentage of body fat. The different editions of the international guidelines of the American Diabetes Association (ADA) highlight the importance of macronutrient consumption and control, however, specific recommendations for micronutrients in diabetes control are limited in the scientific literature [3]. In addition, nutrition is directly related to the success of the anti-hyperglycemic drug therapy of metformin because the absorption of nutrients can influence the pharmacokinetics of the drug and consequently its therapeutic effect [13].

Some studies have explored the relationship between the consumption of macro and micronutrients with the effect of metformin on T2D. Diets high in saturated fat were found to have a negative impact on the effect of metformin on glycemic control

Gene symbol ID	Region	dbSNP ID	SNP	Alleles	Effect	Risk allele				
						AFR	AMR	EAS	EUR	SAS
SLC22A1 6580	6q25.3	rs628031	Missense Met408Val	A/G	↓SE	A 27%	A 22%	A 26%	A 41%	A 39%
		rs12208357	Missense Arg61Cys	C/T	↓	T 0%	T 2%	T 0%	T 6%	T 2%
		rs34130495	Missense Gly401Ser	A/G	↓	A 0%	A 1%	A 0%	A 2%	A 0%
		rs622342	Intronic	C/T	↓	C 18%	C 40%	C 15%	C 38%	C 25%
		rs683369	Missense Leu160Phe	G/C	↓	G 1%	G 11%	G 15%	G 21%	G 17%
		rs36056065	Indel GTAAGTTG	−/GTAAGTTG	SE	ND	ND	ND	ND	ND
		rs594709	Intronic	A/G	↑	G 29%	G 22%	G 26%	G 41%	G 39%
		rs2282143	Missense Pro341Leu	C/T	↑	T 8%	T 2%	T 13%	T 1%	T 8%
		rs72552763	IndelGAT	−/GAT	↓	AT 5%	AT 29%	AT 0%	AT 18%	AT 15%
		rs316019	Missense Ala270Ser	G/T	↓	A 19%	A 9%	A 14%	A 11%	A 13%
		rs145450955	Missense Thr201Met	G/A	↓	A 0%	A 0%	A 1%	A 0%	A 0%
		rs201919874	Missense Thr199Ile	C/T	↓	A 0%	A 0%	A 0%	A 0%	A 0%

ID: Gene ID. dbSNP ID: a unique identifier assigned to a single nucleotide polymorphism (SNP) when it is submitted to the SNP database. Met, Methionine; Val, Valine; Arg, Arginine; Cys, Cysteine; Gly, Glycine; Ser, Serine; Leu, Leucine; Phe, Phenylalanine; Pro, Proline; Ala, Alanine; Thr, Threonine; Ile, Isoleucine. A, Adenine; G, Guanine; C, Cytosine; T, Thymine. ↑, increased response to therapy (in relation to the minor allele); ↓, reduced response to therapy (in relation to the minor allele); SE, side effect. AFR, African; AMR, American; EAS, East Asian; EUR, European; SAS, South Asian.

Table 1.
Genetic variants ton gene SLC22A1 influence metformin therapy outcomes and frequencies by region.

in animal models [38]. Also, it has been reported that the consumption of leucine at doses of 24 g / kg combined with the use of metformin in mice with obesity induced by a high-fat diet, significantly reduced the degree of adiposity, liver weight control, liver, and plasma lipids, as well as inflammatory markers in mice. One of the characteristics of patients with advanced T2D is the accumulation of liver fat and increased dyslipidemias. Therefore, focusing nutritional therapy with combined leucine–metformin intake, even at low doses, appears to have a significant effect on adiposity and completely reverses hepatic steatosis in diet-induced obese mice [39]. The amino acid leucine participates in the activation of the AMPK/Sirt1 signaling pathway, thus modulating energy, lipid, and glycolytic metabolism. Leucine has the ability to activate Sirt1, in part, by reducing energy in NAD+ activation, and as a consequence other sirtuin activators [40]. Also, the combined effect of leucine with resveratrol (nutrient–nutrient interaction) has been evaluated, and increased insulin sensitivity, muscle glucose utilization, and lipid oxidation were found. In this sense, the authors of this study propose the consumption of leucine as an adjuvant amino acid in the efficiency of metformin, since, as this is a drug that also converges in the AMPK/Sirt pathway, the combination of both could be a first-line proposal in patients with T2D, especially those who are overweight or obese [41, 42].

There is increasing evidence that metformin is associated with physiological processes in the gastrointestinal tract, since a pronounced effect can be observed when metformin is administered orally, in that sense, evaluating its interaction with the absorption of specific nutrients from the diet becomes highly relevant within the area of pharmacokinetics [43, 44]. Under this hypothesis, a study in animal models was conducted to evaluate microbiota changes in mice that were fed a high-fat diet and, in addition, received metformin treatment. Stool samples were collected before and after drug treatment and found 100 different species related to metformin. Functional analysis targeting carbohydrate, lipid, and amino acid metabolism pathways revealed 14 modified hierarchies. Sex-specific differences in response to metformin treatment were also observed. Males experienced greater changes in metabolic markers, while females showed important changes in the gut microbiome [45].

Micronutrients such as calcium, magnesium, zinc, potassium, and sodium (Ca, Mg, Zn, K, and Na) are cations that are absorbed in the intestine through the transmembrane channel "transporter of organic cations" (OCT1) mainly. This is the same protein related to the absorption of metformin, so the study of the interactions between the dietary intake of micronutrients with specific variants of the *OCT1* gene in subjects receiving metformin, may explain to some extent the differences in terms of the effect on glycemic control observed in subjects with this pharmacotherapy. A recent study reported that there is a significant interaction between the consumption of specific micronutrients such as calcium and potassium with the risk variant 408*Val* rs628031 of the *SLC22A1/OCT1* gene and glycemic control in T2D patients receiving metformin [13].

With the above, the importance of carrying out Nutrigenetics and Pharmacogenetics studies in patients with T2D is highlighted that allows the timely detection of subjects who do achieve glycemic control based on personalized diet and metformin, while in non-responders seek the particular treatment that guarantees the goal in glycemic control that is HbA1c <7%.

3. Conclusions

The most recognized effect of metformin is the suppression of hepatic glucose production, which favors glycemic control in subjects with TD2. The response to metformin in glycemic control is variable in each population studied, which forces us to study genetic factors related to the pharmacokinetics and pharmacodynamics of this drug to find associated genetic variants that explain these differences to some extent. Metformin is eliminated without structural modification by urine mainly, so genes closely related to its pharmacodynamics such as solute carriers (SLC) are of greatest interest in future studies in Latin America. With the Pharmacogenetics approach, it will be possible to predict the genetic component that differentiated responders from non-responders to drug treatment with metformin for glycemic control in patients with TD2 in Latin America.

The mechanisms of action of metformin are not fully understood, there is evidence of some physiological effects in the intestine that suggest a mechanism in glucose homeostasis and the intestinal microbiome that favors glycemic control in patients with TD2, which makes a promising future of this drug by expanding the target organ.

Interaction studies between metformin and macro or micronutrients with genes encoding organic cation transporters (SLC22), may help improve glycemic control in patients with TD2 from specific populations in Latin America.

Acknowledgements

To the Interinstitutional Program for the Strengthening of Research and Graduate Studies of the Pacific (Dolphin Program) for promoting the collegiate work that led to the creation of the Dolphin Research Networks whiting the mobility subprogram of professors and researchers. To the Board of Trustees to Administer the Special Tax Destined to the Autonomous University of Nayarit, for the support to cover the expenses for Article Processing Charge of this chapter.

Conflict of interest

The authors declare no conflict of interest.

Author details

Eloy A. Zepeda-Carrillo[1*], Rafael Torres Valadez[1,2], Sara A. Campos Huerta[1] and Elisa María Barrón Cabrera[3]

1 Specialized Unit in Research, Development and Innovation in Genomic Medicine, Nayarit Center for Innovation and Technology Transfer, Autonomous University of Nayarit, Tepic, Mexico

2 Integral Health Academic Unit, Autonomous University of Nayarit, Tepic, Mexico

3 Faculty of Nutrition and Gastronomy Sciences, Autonomous University of Sinaloa, Culiacan, Mexico

*Address all correspondence to: eloyz@uan.edu.mx

References

[1] World Health Organization. Global report on diabetes [Internet]. World Health Organization; 2016 [citado 16 de septiembre de 2022]. 83 p. Disponible en: https://apps.who.int/iris/handle/10665/204871

[2] OPS/OMS (Organización Panamericana de la Salud) Diabetes [Internet]. 2016 [citado 16 de septiembre de 2022]. Disponible en: https://www.paho.org/es/temas/diabetes

[3] Inzucchi SE, Bergenstal RM, Buse JB, Diamant M, Ferrannini E, Nauck M, et al. Management of hyperglycemia in type 2 diabetes: a patient-centered approach: Position statement of the American Diabetes Association (ADA) and the European Association for the Study of Diabetes (EASD). Diabetes Care. 2012;**35**(6):1364-1379

[4] He L. Metformin and systemic metabolism. Trends in Pharmacological Sciences. 2020;**41**(11):868-881

[5] Nasykhova YA, Tonyan ZN, Mikhailova AA, Danilova MM, Glotov AS. Pharmacogenetics of type 2 diabetes-progress and prospects. International Journal of Molecular Sciences. 18 de septiembre de 2020;**21**(18):E6842

[6] 1000 Genomes Project Consortium, Auton A, Brooks LD, Durbin RM, Garrison EP, Kang HM, et al. A global reference for human genetic variation. Nature. 1 de octubre de 2015;**526**(7571):68-74

[7] 1000 Genomes Project Consortium, Auton A, Brooks LD, Durbin RM, Garrison EP, Kang HM, et al. A global reference for human genetic variation. rs628031 (SNP). Nature. 1 de octubre de 2015;**526**(7571):68-74

[8] International Diabetes Federation. IDF Diabetes Atlas, 10th edn. Brussels, Belgium. 2021 [citado 22 de septiembre 2022]. Available from: https://www.diabetesatlas.org

[9] International Diabetes Federation. IDF Diabetes Atlas, 10th edn. Brussels, Belgium: International Diabetes Federation; 2021

[10] King H, Aubert RE, Herman WH. Global burden of diabetes, 1995-2025: Prevalence, numerical estimates, and projections. Diabetes Care. 1998;**21**(9):1414-1431

[11] He L, Wondisford FE. Metformin action: Concentrations matter. Cell Metabolism. 3 de febrero de 2015;**21**(2):159-162

[12] Yerevanian A, Soukas AA. Metformin: Mechanisms in human obesity and weight loss. Current Obesity Reports. 2019;**8**(2):156-164

[13] Zepeda-Carrillo EA, Ramos-Lopez O, Martínez-López E, Barrón-Cabrera E, Bernal-Pérez JA, Velasco-González LE, et al. Effect of metformin on glycemic control regarding carriers of the SLC22A1/OCT1 (rs628031) polymorphism and its interactions with dietary micronutrients in type 2 diabetes. DMSO. 2022;**15**:1771-1784

[14] Rena G, Hardie DG, Pearson ER. The mechanisms of action of metformin. Diabetologia. 2017;**60**(9):1577-1585

[15] Hawley SA, Ross FA, Chevtzoff C, Green KA, Evans A, Fogarty S, et al. Use of cells expressing γ subunit variants to identify diverse mechanisms of AMPK activation. Cell Metabolism. 2010;**11**(6):554-565

[16] Wang DS, Jonker JW, Kato Y, Kusuhara H, Schinkel AH, Sugiyama Y. Involvement of organic cation transporter 1 in hepatic and intestinal distribution of metformin. The Journal of Pharmacology and Experimental Therapeutics. 2002;**302**(2):510-515

[17] Bridges HR, Jones AJY, Pollak MN, Hirst J. Effects of metformin and other biguanides on oxidative phosphorylation in mitochondria. The Biochemical Journal 15 de septiembre de 2014;**462**(3):475-487

[18] Fullerton MD, Galic S, Marcinko K, Sikkema S, Pulinilkunnil T, Chen ZP, et al. Single phosphorylation sites in Acc1 and Acc2 regulate lipid homeostasis and the insulin-sensitizing effects of metformin. Nature Medicine. 2013;**19**(12):1649-1654

[19] Pawlyk AC, Giacomini KM, McKeon C, Shuldiner AR, Florez JC. Metformin pharmacogenomics: Current status and future directions. Diabetes. 2014;**63**(8):2590-2599

[20] Foretz M, Guigas B, Bertrand L, Pollak M, Viollet B. Metformin: From mechanisms of action to therapies. Cell Metabolism. 2 de diciembre de 2014;**20**(6):953-966

[21] Miller RA, Chu Q, Xie J, Foretz M, Viollet B, Birnbaum MJ. Biguanides suppress hepatic glucagon signalling by decreasing production of cyclic AMP. Nature. 14 de febrero de 2013;**494**(7436):256-260

[22] Buse JB, DeFronzo RA, Rosenstock J, Kim T, Burns C, Skare S, et al. The primary glucose-lowering effect of metformin resides in the gut, not the circulation: Results from short-term pharmacokinetic and 12-week dose-ranging studies. Diabetes Care. 2016;**39**(2):198-205

[23] Natali A, Ferrannini E. Effects of metformin and thiazolidinediones on suppression of hepatic glucose production and stimulation of glucose uptake in type 2 diabetes: A systematic review. Diabetologia. 2006;**49**(3):434-441

[24] Sundelin E, Gormsen LC, Jensen JB, Vendelbo MH, Jakobsen S, Munk OL, et al. Genetic polymorphisms in organic cation transporter 1 attenuates hepatic metformin exposure in humans. Clinical Pharmacology and Therapeutics. 2017;**102**(5):841-848

[25] Preiss D, Dawed A, Welsh P, Heggie A, Jones AG, Dekker J, et al. Sustained influence of metformin therapy on circulating glucagon-like peptide-1 levels in individuals with and without type 2 diabetes. Diabetes, Obesity and Metabolism. 2017;**19**(3):356-363

[26] Cameron AR, Morrison VL, Levin D, Mohan M, Forteath C, Beall C, et al. Anti-inflammatory effects of metformin irrespective of diabetes status. Circulation Research 19 de agosto de 2016;**119**(5):652-665

[27] Forslund K, Hildebrand F, Nielsen T, Falony G, Le Chatelier E, Sunagawa S, et al. Disentangling type 2 diabetes and metformin treatment signatures in the human gut microbiota. Nature. 10 de diciembre de 2015;**528**(7581):262-266

[28] Zhou K, Bellenguez C, Spencer CCA, Bennett AJ, Coleman RL, Tavendale R, et al. Common variants near ATM are associated with glycemic response to metformin in type 2 diabetes. Nature Genetics. 2011;**43**(2):117-120

[29] Mofo Mato EP, Guewo-Fokeng M, Essop MF, Owira PMO. Genetic polymorphisms of organic cation transporter 1 (OCT1) and responses to metformin therapy in individuals

with type 2 diabetes: A systematic review. Medicine (Baltimore). 2018;**97**(27):e11349

[30] van Leeuwen N, Nijpels G, Becker ML, Deshmukh H, Zhou K, Stricker BHC, et al. A gene variant near ATM is significantly associated with metformin treatment response in type 2 diabetes: A replication and meta-analysis of five cohorts. Diabetologia 1 de julio de 2012;**55**(7):1971-1977

[31] O'Leary NA, Wright MW, Brister JR, Ciufo S, Haddad D, McVeigh R, et al. Reference sequence (RefSeq) database at NCBI: Current status, taxonomic expansion, and functional annotation. Nucleic Acids Res. 4 de enero de 2016;**44**(D1):D733-D745

[32] Zhou K, Yee SW, Seiser EL, van Leeuwen N, Tavendale R, Bennett AJ, et al. Variation in the glucose transporter gene SLC2A2 is associated with glycemic response to metformin. Nature Genetics. 2016;**48**(9):1055-1059

[33] Rathmann W, Strassburger K, Bongaerts B, Kuss O, Müssig K, Burkart V, et al. A variant of the glucose transporter gene SLC2A2 modifies the glycaemic response to metformin therapy in recently diagnosed type 2 diabetes. Diabetologia. 1 de febrero de 2019;**62**(2):286-291

[34] Rotroff DM, Yee SW, Zhou K, Marvel SW, Shah HS, Jack JR, et al. Genetic variants in CPA6 and PRPF31 are associated with variation in response to metformin in individuals with type 2 diabetes. Diabetes. 2018;**67**(7):1428-1440

[35] Tarasova L, Kalnina I, Geldnere K, Bumbure A, Ritenberga R, Nikitina-Zake L, et al. Association of genetic variation in the organic cation transporters OCT1, OCT2 and multidrug and toxin extrusion 1 transporter protein genes with the gastrointestinal side effects and lower BMI in metformin-treated type 2 diabetes patients. Pharmacogenetics and Genomics. 2012;**22**(9):659-666

[36] Florez JC. Pharmacogenetics in type 2 diabetes: Precision medicine or discovery tool? Diabetologia. 1 de mayo de 2017;**60**(5):800-807

[37] 1000 Genomes Project Consortium, Auton A, Brooks LD, Durbin RM, Garrison EP, Kang HM, et al. A global reference for human genetic variation. rs594709 (SNP). Nature. 1 de octubre de 2015;**526**(7571):68-74

[38] Lu X, Dong Y, Jian Z, Li Q, Gong L, Tang L, et al. Systematic investigation of the effects of long-term administration of a high-fat diet on drug transporters in the mouse liver, kidney and intestine. Current Drug Metabolism. 2019;**20**(9):742-755

[39] Fu L, Bruckbauer A, Li F, Cao Q, Cui X, Wu R, et al. Interaction between metformin and leucine in reducing hyperlipidemia and hepatic lipid accumulation in diet-induced obese mice. Metabolism. 2015;**64**(11):1426-1434

[40] Bruckbauer A, Zemel MB. Synergistic effects of polyphenols and methylxanthines with leucine on AMPK/sirtuin-mediated metabolism in muscle cells and adipocytes. PLoS One. 2014;**9**(2):e89166

[41] Kendall DL, Amin R, Clayton PE. Metformin in the treatment of obese children and adolescents at risk of type 2 diabetes. Paediatric Drugs. 2014;**16**(1):13-20

[42] Xu F, Gao Z, Zhang J, Rivera CA, Yin J, Weng J, et al. Lack of SIRT1 (mammalian sirtuin 1) activity leads to liver steatosis in the SIRT1+/− mice:

A role of lipid mobilization and inflammation. Endocrinology. 2010;**151**(6):2504-2514

[43] Wu T, Horowitz M, Rayner CK. New insights into the anti-diabetic actions of metformin: from the liver to the gut. Expert Review of Gastroenterology & Hepatology. 2017;**11**(2):157-166

[44] Stepensky D, Friedman M, Raz I, Hoffman A. Pharmacokinetic-pharmacodynamic analysis of the glucose-lowering effect of metformin in diabetic rats reveals first-pass pharmacodynamic effect. Drug Metabolism and Disposition. 2002;**30**(8):861-868

[45] Silamiķele L, Silamiķelis I, Ustinova M, Kalniņa Z, Elbere I, Petrovska R, et al. Metformin strongly affects gut microbiome composition in high-fat diet-induced type 2 diabetes mouse model of both sexes. Frontiers in Endocrinology (Lausanne). 2021;**12**:626359

Chapter 3

Therapeutic Potential of Metformin in Diabetes Mellitus-Related Cardiovascular Complications

Hongmei Tan and Jun Tao

Abstract

The diabetic population continues to grow worldwide, resulting in many chronic cardiovascular complications, including atherosclerosis and diabetic cardiomyopathy, as well as an increase in the incidence of heart failure. Metformin, as the first-line oral therapy for type 2 diabetes, lowers blood glucose and reduces the incidence of diabetes mellitus (DM)-related cardiovascular events, such as myocardial infarction. The cardiovascular protective effect of metformin is due not only to the relief of insulin resistance and the improvement of glucose and lipid metabolism but also to the inhibition of oxidation and inflammation. Metformin exerts its multiple effects primarily through AMPK-dependent and AMPK-independent mechanisms. This chapter reviews the beneficial effects of metformin on DM-related cardiovascular complications and dissects the potential molecular mechanisms.

Keywords: diabetes mellitus, metformin, cardiovascular complications, AMPK

1. Introduction

Cardiovascular disease (CVD) is the leading cause of death in adults with diabetes mellitus (DM) [1]. DM caused 3.7 million deaths in individuals aged 70 and under, the majority of which were due to cardiovascular disease (43% of this 3.7 million) [2]. According to the action in diabetes and vascular disease: preterax and diamicron modified release controlled evaluation (ADVANCE) trial, adults with diabetes are two to three times more likely than adults without diabetes to develop cardiovascular disease. Adjusted for age at diagnosis, the risk of macrovascular events, including cardiovascular death, nonfatal myocardial infarction, or non-fatal stroke, increased by 49% for each additional 5-year duration of type 2 diabetes in adults. However, more severe hypoglycemic events occurred after intensive glycemic control, and the type of glycemic control had no significant effect on cardiovascular-related mortality [3, 4].

Metformin was not the first blood-glucose-lowering agent to be developed, and the process has an interesting history that begins with the withdrawal of phenformin and buformin (the only other biguanides used to lower blood glucose at that time) after they were found to have harmful effects in clinical trials [5]. Although the evidence

IntechOpen

of cardiovascular benefits was published in the United Kingdom prospective diabetes study (UKPDS) in 1998 [6], metformin emerged as the first-choice and most-prescribed oral medication for lower blood glucose in the USA in 1995 [7]. Recent studies have found that metformin has cardiovascular benefits as well, lowering mortality and morbidity associated with cardiovascular diseases, such as stable coronary artery disease and myocardial infarction [8, 9]. This chapter provides an overview of the cardiovascular benefits of metformin and its underlying mechanisms.

2. Metformin and atherosclerosis (AS)

Over the last 30 years, accumulating evidence has shown that metformin reduces atherosclerotic plaque formation in animals fed a high-cholesterol diet [10, 11]. Metformin significantly reduced atherosclerotic plaque and serum high-sensitivity C-reactive protein while inhibiting the activation of the nuclear factor κ-B (NF-κB) pathway in the vessel wall in a high cholesterol diet-induced atherosclerotic rabbit [11]. The same observation was also made in an atherosclerotic mouse model as well. Metformin treatment decreased plaque formation in a high-cholesterol diet-induced apolipoprotein E knockout ($ApoE^{-/-}$) mouse model [12]. It should be noted that metformin had an effect on plaque instability as well. Recent studies have found that metformin [100 mg/(kg·day)] significantly reduced calcification plaques in $ApoE^{-/-}$ mice fed a high-fat diet (HFD) [13]. These findings suggest that metformin may not only alleviate atherosclerotic plaque formation but also improve plaque stability.

2.1 Metformin and endothelial injury

Vascular endothelial dysfunction is one of the most important pathological alterations and is considered an initial event for the development of AS. Metformin has been shown in clinical studies to improve endothelium-dependent vasodilation in diabetic patients [14]. In a preclinical study, metformin improved nitric oxide (NO)-mediated vasodilation in endothelial cells (ECs) *in vitro* by increasing NO production via the Adenosine 5′-monophosphate (AMP)-activated protein kinase (AMPK) pathway [15, 16]. Dong et al. demonstrated that activating AMPKα2 attenuates endoplasmic reticulum stress in vascular ECs [17], and metformin, an AMPKα2 agonist, protects human coronary artery ECs from diabetic lipoapoptosis by activating AMPK [18].

While investigating the effects of metformin on hyperglycemia and associated insulin resistance, clinical studies have addressed its effects on endothelial dysfunction as well. A study conducted in 2001 on the effects of metformin on endothelial function in type 2 diabetes (T2D) patients demonstrated that metformin improves insulin resistance and endothelium-dependent vasodilation; however, no significant effect of endothelium-independent or nitrate-independent vasodilation was observed in this study [19]. These findings suggest that vasodilatory effects are closely associated with metformin-induced insulin sensitivity. AS is a chronic inflammatory pathological process, and anti-inflammatory therapy is considered a functional approach for alleviating the atherosclerotic process. Long-term treatment (4.3 years) with metformin added to insulin therapy decreased the levels of several inflammatory biomarkers of endothelial dysfunction, such as von Willebrand factor (vWF) and soluble vascular cell adhesion molecule-1 (sVCAM-1) in T2D patients. These data indicate the potential of metformin in reducing cardiovascular events [20].

A similar study was conducted by Vitale et al. in 2005. They recruited 65 patients with metabolic syndrome to investigate the effects of metformin (500 mg, b.i.d, for 3 months) on endothelial function. Metformin treatment increased brachial artery endothelial-dependent flow-mediated dilation. It was shown that insulin resistance and endothelial dysfunction are interrelated and can be affected by metformin [21]. These effects of metformin have been demonstrated to benefit patients with type 1 diabetes as well [22]. In the REMOVAL trial in type 1 diabetes, metformin was shown to reduce cardiovascular risk, but no effect of glycemic control on endothelial dysfunction was observed [23]. Other studies involving women with polycystic ovary syndrome (PCOS) treated with metformin or rosiglitazone have shown that metformin is associated with improved flow-mediated vasodilation and does not affect endothelial relaxation independently, making it more effective than rosiglitazone [24, 25]. Metformin treatment for 3 months improved arterial stiffness and associated endothelial dysfunction and reduced carotid intima-media thickness in women with PCOS [26, 27]. Clinical trials involving metformin monotherapy (NCT00169624) or metformin in combination with other antidiabetic drugs in T2D patients (NCT00169624) and PCOS (NCT01459445) can be found online (https://clinicaltrials.gov). All of the aforementioned findings indicate that metformin monotherapy or in combination with other antidiabetic strategies can be a viable option for treating endothelial dysfunction in patients with hyperglycemia and insulin resistance.

2.1.1 Metformin and inflammatory response in ECs

Metformin (0.1–2.5 μg/ml) has been shown to inhibit advanced glycation end products (AGE)-induced monocyte adhesion by inhibiting endothelial cell adhesion molecules [28]. Metformin (2–10 mM) inhibits tumor necrosis factor (TNF)-α-induced gene expression of vascular cell adhesion molecule 1 (VCAM1), E-selectin, intercellular cell adhesion molecule-1 (ICAM-1), and monocyte chemoattractant protein-1 (MCP-1), thereby facilitating monocyte adhesion to activated ECs and the IKK/IKBα/NF-KB signaling pathway [29]. Poly ADP-ribose polymerase-1 (PARP-1) inhibits the expression of BCL6 (zinc finger protein 51) by binding to its intron 1, and it subsequently increases the expression of pro-inflammatory cytokines, such as VCAM-1 and MCP1. The AMPK activator or metformin (1 mM) induces PARP-1 dissociation from the Bcl-6 intron 1, thereby increasing the expression of Bcl-6, and inhibiting the expression of inflammatory mediators [30]. These findings indicate that metformin may be an effective drug for preventing monocyte adhesion. Additionally, metformin (20 μM) alleviated intracellular oxidative stress by up-regulating the expression of lectin-like oxidized low-density lipoprotein receptor 1 (LOX1) [31].

2.1.2 Metformin and NO production in ECs

NO is crucial for vascular physiological function and maintaining vascular tone. Endothelial nitric oxide synthase (eNOS)-dependent NO production increases endothelium-dependent vasodilation. Metformin (60 mg/kg/d) restores arterial endothelial function in Goto-Kakizaki (GK) rats (a spontaneous T2D animal model) and rats treated with streptozotocin (STZ) (an induced T2D animal model) by increasing NO bioavailability and restoring endothelium-dependent vasodilation [32]. Metformin (50–500 μM) also increases eNOS phosphorylation and its interaction with HSP90, resulting in an increase in NO production. High glucose levels indicate impaired eNOS-HSP90 interaction, which can be restored with metformin [16]. Metformin (250 mg/kg/d) has also been found to activate eNOS in endothelial progenitor cells isolated from STZ-induced diabetic mice [33]. Tetrahydrobiopterin (BH4) is a cofactor for the biological function of eNOS and regulates the NO level, which is important for vascular physiology. Cyclohydrolase 1 (GCH1) is a rate-limiting enzyme in BH4 biosynthesis whose deficiency affects BH4 level. The eNOS-activating effect of metformin is also related to guanosine triphosphate GCH1. Metformin (300 mg/kg/d) increases the protein expression of GCH at a post-translational level [34]. In diabetic and obese mice, this protective effect increases endothelial-dependent vasodilation [35].

2.1.3 Metformin and vascular integrity in ECs

Another leading cause of diabetic vascular change is abnormal vascular integrity. Increased vascular permeability promotes monocyte extravasation. Metformin (0.1–1 mM) has also been shown to decrease vascular permeability of ECs in the brain. Metformin-induced AMPK was demonstrated to be involved in the prevention of endothelial dysfunction [36]. Glycocalyx is a matrix structure that prevents vascular permeability; metformin (0.33 mg/ml) can improve glycocalyx barrier function in db/db mice [37]. Metformin (400 mg/kg, bid) reduced lung endothelial hyperpermeability and systemic inflammatory response by activating AMPK in STZ-induced diabetic mice and db/db diabetic mice. Metformin administration improved survival, which was associated with suppression of VE-cadherin phosphorylation (pVE-cadherin) [38].

2.2 Metformin and macrophage

2.2.1 Metformin and inflammation

Chronic inflammation is an important pathological process in the onset and progression of AS [39]. Cholesterol metabolism homeostasis in macrophages can be disrupted in the process of lipid degradation [40]. The inflammatory response can be activated during the development of AS by free cholesterol (FC), which induces the formation of cholesterol crystals and, subsequently, the formation of foam cells [41]. Excessive chemotaxis retention factors released by foam cells caused pro-inflammatory cytokines and the inflammatory response. Plaque rupture can be caused by excessive inflammation and increases the risk of coronary thrombosis [42]. Currently, targeting cytokines (such as interlukin (IL)-1β, IL-1β; IL-17, and TNF) has been shown to slow the progression of CVD in some cases [43]. Treatment with metformin has been shown to be beneficial in the treatment of macrovascular complications in addition to its hypoglycemic effect. Metformin (0.09 U) can reduce the log-transformed neutrophil to lymphocyte-ratio after 8 to 16 months compared to sulfonylurea therapy. Metformin also inhibited blood cytokines, including the C-C motif chemokine 11 (CCL11) in a non-diabetic heart failure trial (registration: NCT00473876). Methionine increased the levels of homocysteine (Hcy), TNF-α, H_2S, and IL-1β in C57BL/6 mice while decreasing the level of cystathionine g-lyase (CSE). Hcy increased the expression of DNA methyltransferase and the methylation of the CSE promoter in macrophage, whereas metformin treatment can reduce the deleterious effects of methionine [44]. Phosphatase and tensin homolog (PTEN)-deficient macrophages create a persistent inflammatory microenvironment in which they induce nitric oxide synthase (iNOS)/NO and cyclooxygenase-2 (COX)-2/ Prostaglandin E2 (PGE2), which can be inhibited by metformin by inhibiting reactive oxygen species (ROS) production and Akt activation [45]. These anti-inflammatory effects of metformin are also the result of AMPK activation, but even after treatment with compound C, an AMPK inhibitor, residual metformin activity remains significant [46]. Our previous study also demonstrated that metformin inhibits NOD-like receptor thermal protein domain associated protein 3 (NLRP3) inflammasome and suppresses DM-accelerated AS in $ApoE^{-/-}$ mice through AMPK activation [47]. Metformin treatment of mouse or human alveolar macrophages prevents particle-induced production of complex III mitochondrial ROS, thereby inhibiting calcium release-activated channel (CRAC) activation and IL-6 release [48]. These studies suggest that metformin reduces oxidative stress in macrophages.

2.2.2 Metformin and foam cell formation

Foam cells are an important element of atherosclerotic plaque. Macrophages absorb modified plasma-derived lipoproteins, leading to the formation of lipid-filled foam cells and atherosclerotic lesions [39]. Metformin inhibits the accumulation of cholesterol in macrophages under various inducible conditions. The ATP-binding cassette transporter G1 (ABCG1)-mediated cholesterol efflux cannot effectively regulate glycated high-density lipoprotein (HDL) particles. Metformin can restore cholesterol efflux mediated by glycated HDL [49]. This is also observed in oxidized low-density lipoprotein (oxLDL)-stimulated cholesterol accumulation and in foam cell formation, which may be associated with ABCG1 up-regulation. Metformin also reduced the rate of cholesterol biosynthesis from acetate in the J774A.1 macrophage cell line [50]. Metformin inhibits foam cell formation and reduces the expression of adipogenic differentiation-associated protein (ADRP) in LPS-induced THP-1 macrophages [51].

In addition, when metformin is combined with other drugs, its efficacy increases while adverse reactions are reduced. Coadministration of metformin and T317 (liver X receptor agonist) with an HFD alleviated the development of AS in ApoE−/− mice. This was due to a decrease in monocyte adhesion and macrophage cell proliferation, which was associated with an increase in ATP-binding cassette transporter A1(ABCA1)/ ABCG1 expression [52].

2.2.3 Metformin and macrophage polarization

In the pathological process, tissue injury and pro-inflammatory cytokines secretion promote the differentiation of monocytes into macrophages and further exacerbate inflammation [53]. M1 macrophages are traditionally involved in pro-inflammatory and bactericidal activity, whereas M2 macrophages produce anti-inflammatory mediators and growth factors in response to the resolution of inflammation [54]. In a clinical study involving 30 healthy volunteers and 30 obese volunteers (20 with diabetes), the obese volunteers were treated with metformin and peripheral blood mononuclear cells (PBMCs) were isolated to measure polarization markers. The results revealed that the level of the CD68 marker was increased in diabetic patients, while CD11b, CD11c, CD163, and CD169 were decreased. The elevated expression levels of TNF-α, iNOS, IL-6, CD16, CD36, and CD206 indicated the presence of macrophages with an M1-like phenotype. After treatment with metformin, the levels of TNF-α, iNOS, IL-6, CD11c, CD36, CD169, and CD206 showed no significant difference between healthy volunteers and diabetic patients. These results

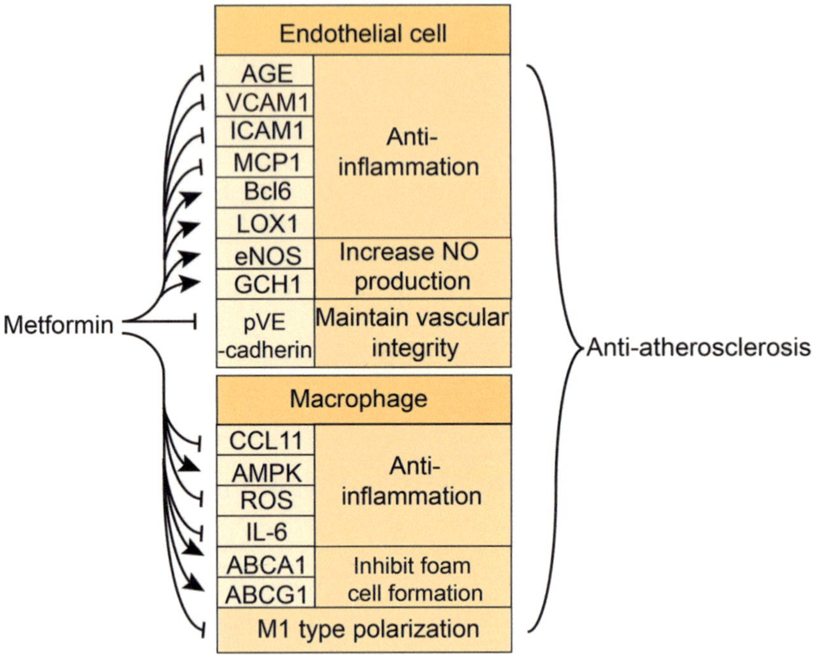

Figure 1.
Schematic of the molecular signaling pathways involved in anti-AS effect of metformin.

suggest a close relationship between metformin treatment and distinct patterns of phenotypic markers [55]. Metformin treatment decreased not only M1 macrophage marker levels (MCP1 and CD11c) but also blood levels of TNF-α and IL-6 in male C57/6 J mice fed an HFD for 7 weeks. Therefore, metformin-regulated AMPK may be involved in M2 phenotype macrophages and decreases inflammation in obesity [56]. Chronic metformin administration also promoted microglia/macrophage M2 polarization by regulating AMPK, which may improve functional recovery after middle cerebral artery occlusion (MCAO) in mice [57]. Metformin-activated AMPK also induced macrophage M2 polarization and inflammatory cytokines expression, alleviating the formation of atherosclerotic plaque [57].

Taken together, metformin has been shown to have a great anti-AS effect by regulating different molecular signaling pathways related to vascular homeostases, such as increasing NO production, maintaining endothelial integrity, decreasing oxidative stress, preventing M1 type polarization, inhibiting inflammation, and so on (**Figure 1**).

3. Metformin and diabetic cardiomyopathy

Diabetic cardiomyopathy (DCM) is typically characterized by left ventricular (LV) dysfunction and the absence of a history of coronary artery disease or hypertension [58, 59]. The molecular mechanism initiating DCM is unclear, but the major clinical and biochemical dysfunctions in DCM development have been identified, such as hyperglycemia, systemic insulin resistance, and impaired cardiac insulin signaling [60–62]. Emerging evidence highlights the significance of abnormal mitochondrial function and energy metabolism in causing pathological remodeling of the cardiac structure [63, 64].

Metformin has been shown to be cardioprotective in ongoing clinical and basic research and it has been recommended as first-line therapy in diabetic patients with heart failure (HF) based on clinical practice guidelines [65]. Numerous studies have shown that monotherapy or combination therapy with metformin reduces mortality and/or hospitalizations in patients with diabetes and/or HF [66]. Similarly, a 10-year follow-up study revealed that metformin reduced the incidence of myocardial infarction from all causes [67]. In basic research, it was found that metformin protects against oxidative stress [68, 69]. It attenuates pro-inflammatory responses induced by LPS or oxidative stress [70, 71]. However, there are contradictory analyses of these positive reports as well [72, 73].

3.1 Metformin and free fatty acid (FFA) metabolism

In diabetic patients, increasing FFA released from adipose tissue leads to an increase in circulating levels, especially in patients with visceral adiposity. Abnormal circulating levels of FFAs cause a shift from glucose to FFA uptake and utilization, impairing myocardial energy metabolism [74, 75]. This elevated FFA in circulation also increases the expression of the nuclear receptor peroxisome proliferator-activated receptor-α (PPAR-α) [76]. Activated PPAR-α improves the expression of FFA oxidation-related genes (pyruvate dehydrogenase kinase 4, PDK4; CD36), thereby increasing mitochondrial FFA uptake [77]. Myocardial FFA uptake that exceeds its FFA β-oxidation capacity results in lipid accumulation [78]. This metabolic disorder protects against subsequent oxidation and toxic lipid metabolites at first, but this metabolic imbalance eventually leads to mechanical dysfunction and organ failure. Lipid accumulation also promotes the production of toxic lipid intermediates (diacylglycerol, DAG; ceramides) which contribute to oxidative stress and cardiomyocyte apoptosis. Research has shown that lipid accumulation in myocytes is closely related to the severity of ischemia–reperfusion (IR) and CVD [79, 80].

Metformin treatment was associated with a decrease in fasting plasma glucose ($P < 0.05$), insulin ($P < 0.05$), triglyceride [TG] ($P < 0.05$), and FFA ($P < 0.03$) levels, according to a 2004 study involving 120 overweight T2D patients treated with placebo + diet ($n = 60$) or metformin (850 mg twice daily) + diet ($n = 60$) for 4 months [81]. Jeppesen also demonstrated that metformin treatment lowers postprandial glucose, insulin, FFA, and TG levels ($P < 0.001$) in patients with non-insulin-dependent DM (NIDDM) [82]. During the early stages of hypertension, spontaneously hypertensive rats (SHR) exhibited myocardial metabolic changes including FFA. Metformin-treated SHR exhibited normalization of FFA levels, mean arterial blood pressure, cardiac glucose uptake rates, left ventricular mass/tibia length, and wall thickness. Metformin may exert its effects mechanically by increasing fatty acid oxidation and decreasing oxidative stress by activating AMPK [83]. These findings suggest that the cardioprotective effect of metformin is attributable to its ability to lower FFA levels.

3.2 Metformin and AGE

The nonenzymatic glycation and oxidation of proteins and lipids result in the formation of AGE, and this is an important pathogenetic change in DCM [84]. AGE can covalently bind to each other or to extracellular proteins, such as collagen, laminin, and elastin, rendering the AGE complex vulnerable [84]. This can impair the degradation of collagen leading to collagen accumulation and fibrosis, which causes local tissue stiffness and increases myocardial stiffness [85].

In a clinical trial, metformin (1700 mg daily) was administered to 15 T2D patients for 3 months; the results indicated that patients treated with metformin had lower levels of circulating AGE, which was associated with fasting plasma glucose and glycated hemoglobin after 3 months of treatment [86]. Although the exact molecular mechanism is unknown, metformin is thought to bind its guanidine group to the α-dicarbonyl group of methylglyoxal, which is an intermediate in the formation of AGE, leading to the neutralization of reactive dicarbonyls. Furthermore, metformin activates glyoxolase, promoting the conversion of methylglyoxal to D-lactate [87, 88].

3.3 Metformin and mitochondrial dysfunction

The heart is an energy-dependent organ with abundant mitochondria that provide cellular energy through oxidative phosphorylation. In a diabetic model, abnormal dynamic mitochondrial structure was observed, as well as impaired function and decreased glutathione concentration in mitochondria, all of which promote DCM [89]. On the other hand, proteomic research proteins from mouse cardiomyocytes of the type 1 diabetes model revealed that a large portion of the altered proteins was related to mitochondrial origin and FFA oxidation [90]. This decrease in mitochondrial respiration and expression of the proteins involved in oxidative phosphorylation was also observed in an obese T2D mouse model, suggesting that impaired mitochondrial oxidative capacity and reduced ATP production promote cardiac dysfunction and subsequently limit myocardial contractility [91]. A recent study by Anderson et al. indicates that reducing mitochondrial dysfunction and oxidative stress in diabetic patients may promote the pathogenesis of HF [92].

Metformin has been reported to have a potent effect on improving mitochondria function and regulating the metabolism of cardiomyocytes in a failing heart. Metformin-induced activation of AMPK upregulated the expression of eNOS and peroxisome proliferator-activated receptor-gamma coactivator 1-alpha (PGC-1α), which are important in regulating the biogenesis and function of mitochondria [93, 94]. Metformin increased the expression of stimulated NADH dehydrogenase (ubiquinone) alpha subcomplex-1 (NDUFA1), NDUFA2, NDUFA13, and manganese superoxide dismutase, indicating that it promotes mitochondrial biogenesis under hyperglycemic conditions, as well as mitochondrial biogenesis-related transcription factors (nuclear respiratory factor; NRF-1 and NRF-2). Metformin also upregulated mitochondrial NDUFA13 protein expression by activating AMPK signaling [95].

3.4 Metformin and oxidative stress

The intracellular imbalance between ROS production and antioxidant regulation leads to oxidative stress. The pathological process in both type 1 and type 2 rodent diabetic models is associated with excessive ROS production in the mitochondria [96]. Increased ROS production from both non-mitochondrial (activating NADPH oxidase) and mitochondrial (modulating mitochondrial electron chain to generate superoxide) sources as a result of various risk factors may lead to cardiac dysfunction by directly damaging proteins or DNA or inducing apoptosis [97]. It is notable that a reaction between ROS and NO produces peroxynitrite species, which triggers a range of pathogenic events including impaired coagulation and inflammation [98]. The progression of oxidative damage and antioxidant defect leads to a number of responses that promote ventricular remodeling, including cardiomyocyte hypertrophy [99, 100].

Metformin has been studied for its antioxidative capacity in animal models. Previously, activation of protein phosphatase 2A (PP2A) was shown to attenuate myocardial cell apoptosis *in vitro* under high glucose conditions by deactivating NF-κB signaling [101]. Metformin has been shown to reduce ROS production, pro-inflammatory mediator release, and NF-κB signaling in human and rat primary cardiomyocytes in response to high glucose levels by activating PP2A [102]. Metformin has been reported to prevent mitochondrial dysfunction, alleviate intracellular oxidative stress, and prevent the loss of aconitase activity that was linked to the development of diabetes in the aorta and kidney of Goto-Kakizaki rats. However, this effect was not observed in the heart during hyperglycemia or after administration of metformin [103].

3.5 Metformin and calcium homeostasis

Ca^{2+} in cardiomyocytes is a crucial regulator of cardiac contractility. Diabetic myocytes exhibited abnormal protein modifications, including a shift in myosin isoenzyme composition (from V1 to V3 isoforms) and an abnormal predominance of the β myosin heavy chain (MHC), which resulted in a decrease in contractile protein Ca-ATPase activity and shortening velocity [104]. The diabetic heart was also observed to have abnormal intracellular Ca^{2+} handling during the contractile cycle, as a result of ryanodine receptor-mediated Ca^{2+} release reduction from the sarcoplasmic reticulum (SR) and a decrease in the upstroke phase of the Ca^{2+} transient in streptozotocin-induced diabetic rats. This may result in cardiac dysfunction [105]. Ca^{2+} dysregulation was determined in human cardiomyocytes from T2D patients, and decreased Ca^{2+} sensitivity in myofilaments was observed [106]. The sarco- (endo-) plasmic reticulum Ca^{2+} ATPase (SERCA) 2 is a key enzyme in the regulation of Ca^{2+} localization in SR and has a close relationship with contractile dysfunction. Decreased activity of SERCA was observed in cardiomyocytes incubated in high-glucose medium, in which abnormal Ca^{2+} signaling has been reported [107]. There is also a hypothesis that the slower transient Ca^{2+} kinetics in the diabetic heart results from a slower action potential and reduced SERCA2a expression [108]. The dysfunctional calcium homeostasis and its clinical consequences require further confirmation.

Metformin was reported to have a novel therapeutic perspective role in regulating abnormal mitochondrial Ca^{2+} content in dystrophin-deficient mice, which is a mitochondrial dysfunction model, and mitochondrial Ca^{2+} uptake kinetics significantly increased the mitochondrial Ca^{2+} content. In metformin-treated cardiomyocytes from 3-month-old dystrophin-deficient mice, decreased mitochondrial Ca^{2+} content and

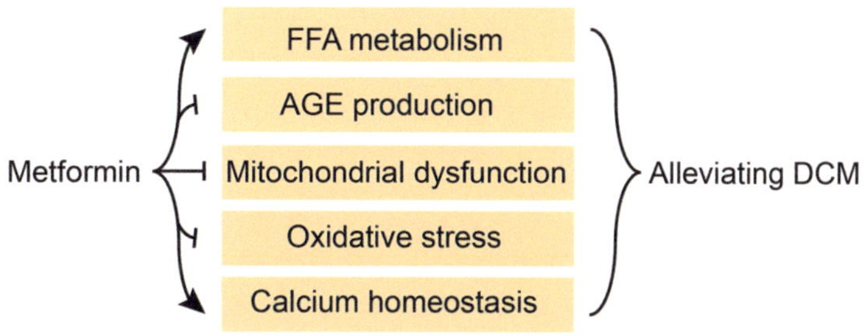

Figure 2.
Schematic of the cardioprotective mechanisms of metformin on DCM.

increased complex I-driven respiration were observed [109]. However, there is no direct evidence that metformin regulates Ca^{2+} homeostasis in cardiomyocytes.

In conclusion, Metformin alleviates DCM development in different approaches, such as promoting FFA oxidation, decreasing FFA and AGE levels, reducing toxic lipid metabolite, and protecting against oxidative damage (**Figure 2**).

4. Metformin and cardiac ischemia: Reperfusion injury

In 1998, the UKPDS study reported that metformin treatment was associated with a 39% reduction in the risk of myocardial infarction (MI), and a 36% and 42% reduction, respectively, in 10-year overall mortality and diabetes-related mortality, compared to insulin or sulfonylureas (SUDs) therapy [6, 67, 110]. According to data from the reduction of atherothrombosis for continued health registry, metformin use is associated with a 24% reduction in all-cause mortality [111]. In a meta-analysis of observational studies, Pladevall et al. found that metformin is associated with a lower risk of MI when compared to SUDs [112]. In the rat models of MI, metformin administration was found to reduce infarct size, preserve myocardial function, and attenuate myocardial remodeling [113, 114].

In a study conducted in 1988, it was demonstrated that oral administration of metformin reduces infarct size 48 h after coronary artery ligation in a mammalian model [115, 116]. Solskov et al. found that a single dose of metformin (250 mg/kg, orally) 24 h before coronary occlusion reduced infarct size in the Langen-dorff isolated rat heart perfused model [113]. Research has shown that a much lower dose of metformin (125 ug/kg) administered intraperitoneal 18 h before ischemia reduced infarct size by more than 50% [117]. In the other isolated working rat heart model, metformin treatment appeared to promote the recovery of contractile function before ischemia and during reperfusion. This finding reflects an effect on cardiac pumping [118].

Clinical and animal studies have shown that metformin has an effective role in ischemia–reperfusion injury, and mechanical studies have provided a new perspective on metformin. Calvert et al. reported that phosphorylation of AMPK occurs after the onset of myocardial ischemia and remains active for 24 hours or more following reperfusion in a murine model of coronary artery occlusion. In rat hearts exposed or not to ischemia, a very low dose of metformin augmented the phosphorylation of AMPK. This implies that the beneficial effect of metformin on ischemia–reperfusion injury is AMPK-dependent. Recent research has shown that metformin-induced eNOS phosphorylation activates AMPK, which is also required for cardioprotective action [117, 119]. One of the first things that happen is mitochondrial dysfunction, which leads to regulated cell death, oxidative stress, and the release of inflammatory cytokines. Mitochondrial dysfunction is caused by an abnormal opening of the mitochondrial permeability transition pore (mPTP), which is also seen in ischemia–reperfusion injury. Immediately after reperfusion, the mPTP opening causes the release of pro-apoptotic factors, such as cytochrome C [120, 121]. It has been reported that metformin activates several kinases of the Reperfusion Injury Salvage Kinase (RISK) pathway like phosphatidylinositol-3-kinase (PI3K) and Akt, thereby restoring abnormal opening of the mPTP (**Figure 3**). In a mammalian study (nondiabetic Wistar rats and type 2 diabetic Goto-Kakizaki rats), metformin upregulated the level of Akt phosphorylation after reperfusion, while concurrent administration of a PI3K inhibitor prevented Akt phosphorylation and abrogated the protective effect of metformin [122].

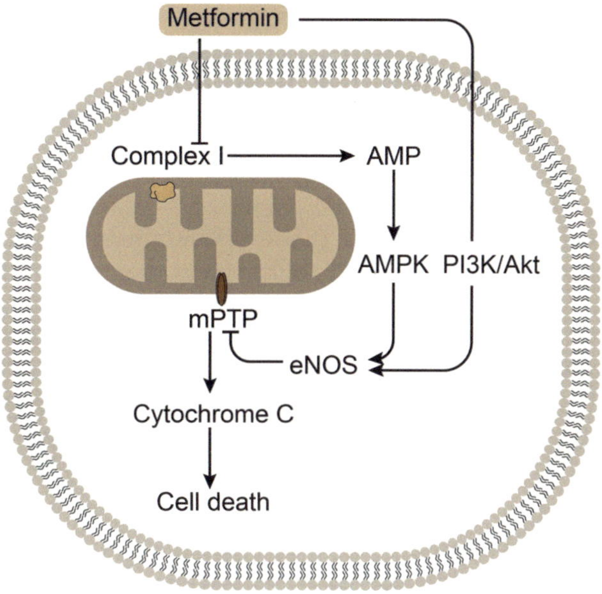

Figure 3.
Schematic of the signaling pathways of metformin in regulating eNOS level and mPTP.

5. Metformin and heart failure

The therapeutic effects of metformin in HF appear beneficial based on clinical trials, as it reduces all-cause mortality and improves cardiac function, as confirmed by the American diabetes association [65]. In an observational study involving 10,920 HF patients taking metformin, sulfonylureas, and/or insulin, the sulfonylurea monotherapy group served as a reference group. This study demonstrated that metformin in monotherapy and in combination with sulfonylureas was associated with a reduction in all-cause mortality compared to sulfonylureas in monotherapy; These findings were consistent with those of a separate analysis of patients treated with or without insulin [72]. Another observational study involved 16,417 T2D patients discharged with a major diagnosis of HF. These patients were treated with thiazolidinediones (n = 2226), metformin (n = 1861), or both thiazolidinediones and metformin (n = 261). Although patients treated with metformin had a lower risk of hospitalization for HF, there was no significant difference in all-cause hospitalization between the three groups [9]. In an analysis of the PL-ASC registry (Polish registry of acute coronary syndromes), admitted diabetic patients with acute coronary syndrome who underwent percutaneous coronary intervention (PCI) were accessed. Two groups of patients were compared: those who used metformin and those who did not. Therefore, metformin treatment has been shown to benefit HF patients and discharges [123].

In vivo or *in vitro* basic research also determined the therapeutic role of metformin in cardiomyopathy, which may lead to HF progression. Metformin has been reported as an anti-inflammatory agent and an antioxidant in cardiomyopathy via AMPK-dependent and AMPK-independent mechanisms. Metformin inhibited high glucose-induced oxidative stress in H9C2 cardiomyocytes by promoting mitochondrial biogenesis, mitochondrial biogenesis-related transcription factors, and AMPK activation [95]. Yang et al. demonstrated that metformin improved diabetic heart function by inhibiting the NLRP3 inflammasome; however, AMPK inhibitors can counteract this effect. Furthermore, metformin inhibited NLRP3 inflammasome-induced cell death by inhibiting mTOR and promoting autophagy [124]. Lai et al. established the 2-hit pulmonary hypertension associated with heart failure with preserved ejection fraction (PH-HFpEF) model (double-leptin receptor defect (obese ZSF1) with the combined treatment of vascular endothelial growth factor receptor blocker SU5416) in rats with multiple features of metabolic syndrome. The glucose-lowering effect of the agent was abrogated in Sirtuin3 (SIRT3)-deficient human skeletal muscle cells and in SIRT3 knockout mice fed an HFD. Additionally, oral metformin treatment on model rats reduced right ventricular systolic pressure and media well thickness, which was associated with activated AMPK and SIRT3 levels. These findings indicate that metformin normalizes PH-HFpEF in a rat model involving AMPK and SIRT3 activation [125]. Hence, these findings demonstrated the role of metformin diabetic cardiomyopathy.

6. Conclusion

Over the course of 50 years of clinical experience, metformin has been well-established as the first-line hypoglycemic drug for the management of diabetes. Metformin inhibits hepatic gluconeogenesis to exert its antihyperglycemic effect. Metformin inhibits the respiratory-chain complex 1, resulting in a decrease in energy charge and a subsequent reduction in hepatic glucose output. These lipid-lowering effects and improvements in insulin sensitivity are primarily dependent on the AMPK signaling pathway.

It is evident that metformin plays a significant role in diabetic cardiomyopathy at various sites. Metformin promotes FFA oxidation and decreases FFA levels, thereby preventing oxidative stress and toxic lipid metabolites. Metformin decreases AGE levels and may alleviate collagen accumulation and fibrosis, which subsequently reduces myocardial stiffness. Importantly, metformin restores mitochondrial function, decreasing intracellular ROS levels and oxidative stress. The chronic administration of metformin to patients has cardioprotective effects, reducing the risk of heart failure and myocardial ischemia–reperfusion injury. Various molecular mechanisms are implicated in the beneficial effects of metformin, such as reducing oxidative stress and cell death via AMPK-dependent and AMPK-independent pathways. Metformin influences vascular physiology by increasing NO production, maintaining endothelial integrity, decreasing oxidative stress, and inhibiting inflammation, all of which contribute to its anti-AS effect. Metformin is regarded by clinicians as an established drug with a significant role in the treatment of T2D. However, there are still many significant unanswered questions from a mechanistic perspective. Understanding the pharmacological mechanisms of metformin may aid in the treatment of not only diabetes but also cardiovascular diseases.

Acknowledgements

This work was supported by the National Natural Science Foundation of China (grant numbers 81873514 and 82170357) and Natural Science Foundation of Guangdong province (grant numbers 2021A1515011766).

Conflict of interest

The authors declare no conflict of interest.

Author details

Hongmei Tan* and Jun Tao
Department of Pathophysiology, School of Medicine, Sun Yat-sen University, Shenzhen, China

*Address all correspondence to: tanhm@mail.sysu.edu.cn

References

[1] The Emerging Risk Factors, C. Diabetes mellitus, fasting blood glucose concentration, and risk of vascular disease: A collaborative meta-analysis of 102 prospective studies. The Lancet. 2010;**375**:2215-2222

[2] Sheet, W.H.O.D.F. Global report on diabetes. 2016

[3] Patel A, MacMahon S, et al. Intensive blood glucose control and vascular outcomes in patients with type 2 diabetes. The New England Journal of Medicine. 2008;**358**:2560-2572

[4] Zoungas S, Woodward M, Li Q, et al. Impact of age, age at diagnosis and duration of diabetes on the risk of macrovascular and microvascular complications and death in type 2 diabetes. Diabetologia. 2014;**57**:2465-2474

[5] Seltzer HS. A summary of criticisms of the findings and conclusions of the university group diabetes program (UGDP). Diabetes. 1972;**21**:976-979

[6] Group, U. Effect of intensive blood-glucose control with metformin on complications in overweight patients with type 2 diabetes (UKPDS 34). Lancet. 1998;**352**:854-865

[7] Bailey CJ. Metformin: Historical overview. Diabetologia. 2017;**60**:1566-1576

[8] Eurich DT, Weir DL, Majumdar SR, et al. Comparative safety and effectiveness of metformin in patients with diabetes mellitus and heart failure: Systematic review of observational studies involving 34,000 patients. Circulation. Heart Failure. 2013;**6**:395-402

[9] Masoudi FA, Inzucchi SE, Wang Y, et al. Thiazolidinediones, metformin, and outcomes in older patients with diabetes and heart failure: An observational study. Circulation. 2005;**5**:583-590

[10] Sirtori CR, Catapano A, Ghiselli GC, et al. Metformin: An antiatherosclerotic agent modifying very low density lipoproteins in rabbits. Atherosclerosis. 1977;**26**:79-89

[11] Li SN, Wang X, Zeng QT, et al. Metformin inhibits nuclear factor kappaB activation and decreases serum high-sensitivity C-reactive protein level in experimental atherogenesis of rabbits. Heart and Vessels. 2009;**24**:446-453

[12] Forouzandeh F, Salazar G, Patrushev N, et al. Metformin beyond diabetes: Pleiotropic benefits of metformin in attenuation of atherosclerosis. Journal of the American Heart Association. 2014;**3**:e001202

[13] Cai Z, Ding Y, Zhang M, et al. Ablation of adenosine monophosphate-activated protein kinase alpha1 in vascular smooth muscle cells promotes diet-induced atherosclerotic calcification In vivo. Circulation Research. 2016;**119**:422-433

[14] de Aguiar LG, Bahia LR, Villela N, et al. Metformin improves endothelial vascular reactivity in first-degree relatives of type 2 diabetic patients with metabolic syndrome and normal glucose tolerance. Diabetes Care. 2006;**29**:1083-1089

[15] O'Hora TR, Markos F, Wiernsperger NF, et al. Metformin causes nitric oxide-mediated dilatation in a shorter time than insulin in the iliac

artery of the anesthetized pig. Journal of Cardiovascular Pharmacology. 2012;**59**:182-187

[16] Davis BJ, Xie Z, Viollet B, et al. Activation of the AMP-activated kinase by antidiabetes drug metformin stimulates nitric oxide synthesis in vivo by promoting the association of heat shock protein 90 and endothelial nitric oxide synthase. Diabetes. 2006;**55**:496-505

[17] Dong Y, Zhang M, Liang B, et al. Reduction of AMP-activated protein kinase alpha2 increases endoplasmic reticulum stress and atherosclerosis in vivo. Circulation. 2010;**121**:792-803

[18] Eriksson L, Nystrom T. Activation of AMP-activated protein kinase by metformin protects human coronary artery endothelial cells against diabetic lipoapoptosis. Cardiovascular Diabetology. 2014;**13**:152

[19] Mather KJ, Verma S, Anderson TJ. Improved endothelial function with metformin in type 2 diabetes mellitus. Journal of the American College of Cardiology. 2001;**37**:1344-1350

[20] de Jager J, Kooy A, Schalkwijk C, et al. Long-term effects of metformin on endothelial function in type 2 diabetes: A randomized controlled trial. Journal of Internal Medicine. 2014;**275**:59-70

[21] Vitale C, Mercuro G, Cornoldi A, et al. Metformin improves endothelial function in patients with metabolic syndrome. Journal of Internal Medicine. 2005;**258**:250-256

[22] Pitocco D, Zaccardi F, Tarzia P, et al. Metformin improves endothelial function in type 1 diabetic subjects: A pilot, placebo-controlled randomized study. Diabetes, Obesity & Metabolism. 2013;**15**:427-431

[23] Petrie JR, Chaturvedi N, Ford I, et al. Cardiovascular and metabolic effects of metformin in patients with type 1 diabetes (REMOVAL): A double-blind, randomised, placebo-controlled trial. The Lancet Diabetes and Endocrinology. 2017;**5**:597-609

[24] Jensterle M, Sebestjen M, Janez A, et al. Improvement of endothelial function with metformin and rosiglitazone treatment in women with polycystic ovary syndrome. European Journal of Endocrinology. 2008;**159**:399-406

[25] Naka KK, Kalantaridou SN, Kravariti M, et al. Effect of the insulin sensitizers metformin and pioglitazone on endothelial function in young women with polycystic ovary syndrome: A prospective randomized study. Fertility and Sterility. 2011;**95**:203-209

[26] Agarwal N, Rice SP, Bolusani H, et al. Metformin reduces arterial stiffness and improves endothelial function in young women with polycystic ovary syndrome: A randomized, placebo-controlled, crossover trial. The Journal of Clinical Endocrinology and Metabolism. 2010;**95**:722-730

[27] Kaya MG, Yildirim S, Calapkorur B, et al. Metformin improves endothelial function and carotid intima media thickness in patients with PCOS. Gynecological Endocrinology. 2015;**31**:401-405

[28] Mamputu JC, Wiernsperger N, Renier G. Metformin inhibits monocyte adhesion to endothelial cells and foam cell formation. The. British Journal of Diabetes & Vascular Disease. 2003;**3**:302-310

[29] Hattori Y, Suzuki K, Hattori S, et al. Metformin inhibits cytokine-induced nuclear factor kappaB activation

via AMP-activated protein kinase activation in vascular endothelial cells. Hypertension. 2006;**47**:1183-1188

[30] Gongol B, Marin T, Peng IC, et al. AMPKalpha2 exerts its anti-inflammatory effects through PARP-1 and Bcl-6. Proceedings of the National Academy of Sciences of the United States of America. 2013;**110**:3161-3166

[31] Hung CH, Chan SH, Chu PM, et al. Metformin regulates oxLDL-facilitated endothelial dysfunction by modulation of SIRT1 through repressing LOX-1-modulated oxidative signaling. Oncotarget. 2016;**7**:10773-10787

[32] Sena CM, Matafome P, Louro T, et al. Metformin restores endothelial function in aorta of diabetic rats. British Journal of Pharmacology. 2011;**163**:424-437

[33] Yu JW, Deng YP, Han X, et al. Metformin improves the angiogenic functions of endothelial progenitor cells via activating AMPK/eNOS pathway in diabetic mice. Cardiovascular Diabetology. 2016;**15**:88

[34] Kidokoro K, Satoh M, Channon KM, et al. Maintenance of endothelial guanosine triphosphate cyclohydrolase I ameliorates diabetic nephropathy. Journal of American Society Nephrology. 2013;**24**:1139-1150

[35] Cheang WS, Tian XY, Wong WT, et al. Metformin protects endothelial function in diet-induced obese mice by inhibition of endoplasmic reticulum stress through 5′ adenosine monophosphate-activated protein kinase-peroxisome proliferator-activated receptor delta pathway. Arteriosclerosis Thrombosis and Vascular Biology. 2014;**34**:830-836

[36] Takata F, Dohgu S, Matsumoto J, et al. Metformin induces up-regulation of blood-brain barrier functions by activating AMP-activated protein kinase in rat brain microvascular endothelial cells. Biochemical and Biophysical Research Communications. 2013;**433**:586-590

[37] Eskens BJ, Zuurbier CJ, van Haare J, et al. Effects of two weeks of metformin treatment on whole-body glycocalyx barrier properties in db/db mice. Cardiovascular Diabetology. 2013;**12**:175

[38] Yang Y, Dong R, Hu D, et al. Liver kinase B1/AMP-activated protein kinase pathway activation attenuated the progression of endotoxemia in the diabetic mice. Cellular Physiology and Biochemistry. 2017;**42**:761-779

[39] Back M, Yurdagul A Jr, Tabas I, et al. Inflammation and its resolution in atherosclerosis: Mediators and therapeutic opportunities. Nature Reviews. Cardiology. 2019;**16**:389-406

[40] Wang D, Yang Y, Lei Y, et al. Targeting foam cell formation in atherosclerosis: Therapeutic potential of natural products. Pharmacological Reviews. 2019;**71**:596-670

[41] Moore KJ, Sheedy FJ, Fisher EA. Macrophages in atherosclerosis: A dynamic balance. Nature Reviews. Immunology. 2013;**13**:709-721

[42] Cameron AR, Morrison VL, Levin D, et al. Anti-inflammatory effects of metformin irrespective of diabetes status. Circulation Research. 2016;**119**:652-665

[43] Williams JW, Huang LH, Randolph GJ. Cytokine circuits in cardiovascular disease. Immunity. 2019;**50**:941-954

[44] Ma X, Jiang Z, Wang Z, et al. Administration of metformin alleviates

atherosclerosis by promoting H2S production via regulating CSE expression. Journal of Cellular Physiology. 2020;**235**:2102-2112

[45] Lin CF, Young KC, Bai CH, et al. Blockade of reactive oxygen species and Akt activation is critical for anti-inflammation and growth inhibition of metformin in phosphatase and tensin homolog-deficient RAW264.7 cells. Immunopharmacology and Immunotoxicology. 2013;**35**:669-677

[46] Buldak L, Labuzek K, Buldak RJ, et al. Metformin affects macrophages' phenotype and improves the activity of glutathione peroxidase, superoxide dismutase, catalase and decreases malondialdehyde concentration in a partially AMPK-independent manner in LPS-stimulated human monocytes/macrophages. Pharmacological Reports. 2014;**66**:418-429

[47] Tang G, Duan F, Li W, et al. Metformin inhibited nod-like receptor protein 3 inflammasomes activation and suppressed diabetes-accelerated atherosclerosis in apoE(−/−) mice. Biomedicine & Pharmacotherapy. 2019;**119**:109410

[48] Soberanes S, Misharin AV, Jairaman A, et al. Metformin targets mitochondrial Electron transport to reduce air-pollution-induced thrombosis. Cell Metabolism. 2019;**29**:335-347

[49] Matsuki K, Tamasawa N, Yamashita M, et al. Metformin restores impaired HDL-mediated cholesterol efflux due to glycation. Atherosclerosis. 2009;**206**:434-438

[50] Koren-Gluzer M, Aviram M, Hayek T. Metformin inhibits macrophage cholesterol biosynthesis rate: Possible role for metformin-induced oxidative stress. Biochemical and Biophysical Research Communications. 2013;**439**:396-400

[51] Xie Z, Yuan Y, Shi J, et al. Metformin Inhibits THP-1 Macrophage-Derived Foam Cell Formation Induced by Lipopolysaccharide. Xi Bao Yu Fen Zi Mian Yi Xue Za Zhi. 2016;**32**:168-172

[52] Ma C, Zhang W, Yang X, et al. Functional interplay between liver X receptor and AMP-activated protein kinase alpha inhibits atherosclerosis in apolipoprotein E-deficient mice - a new anti-atherogenic strategy. British Journal of Pharmacology. 2018;**175**:1486-1503

[53] Tesch GH. Role of macrophages in complications of type 2 diabetes. Clinical and Experimental Pharmacology & Physiology. 2007;**34**:1016-1019

[54] Riabov V, Gudima A, Wang N, et al. Role of tumor associated macrophages in tumor angiogenesis and lymphangiogenesis. Frontiers in Physiology. 2014;**5**:75

[55] Al Dubayee MS, Alayed H, Almansour R, et al. Differential expression of human peripheral mononuclear cells phenotype markers in type 2 diabetic patients and type 2 diabetic patients on metformin. Frontier in Endocrinology (Lausanne). 2018;**9**:537

[56] Jing Y, Wu F, Li D, et al. Metformin improves obesity-associated inflammation by altering macrophages polarization. Molecular and Cellular Endocrinology. 2018;**461**:256-264

[57] Jin Q, Cheng J, Liu Y, et al. Improvement of functional recovery by chronic metformin treatment is associated with enhanced alternative activation of microglia/macrophages and increased angiogenesis and neurogenesis following experimental

stroke. Brain, Behavior, and Immunity. 2014;**40**:131-142

[58] Jia G, Hill MA, Sowers JR. Diabetic cardiomyopathy: An update of mechanisms contributing to this clinical entity. Circulation Research. 2018;**122**:624-638

[59] Nakamura M, Sadoshima J. Cardiomyopathy in obesity, insulin resistance and diabetes. The Journal of Physiology. 2020;**598**:2977-2993

[60] Chong CR, Clarke K, Levelt E. Metabolic Remodeling in diabetic cardiomyopathy. Cardiovascular Research. 2017;**113**:422-430

[61] Boudina S, Abel ED. Diabetic cardiomyopathy revisited. Circulation. 2007;**115**:3213-3233

[62] Sung MM, Hamza SM, Dyck JR. Myocardial metabolism in diabetic cardiomyopathy: Potential therapeutic targets. Antioxidants & Redox Signaling. 2015;**22**:1606-1630

[63] Perseghin G, Ntali G, De Cobelli F, et al. Abnormal left ventricular energy metabolism in obese men with preserved systolic and diastolic functions is associated with insulin resistance. Diabetes Care. 2007;**30**:1520-1526

[64] Ye H, He Y, Zheng C, et al. Type 2 diabetes complicated with heart failure: Research on therapeutic mechanism and potential drug development based on insulin Signaling pathway. Frontiers in Pharmacology. 2022;**13**:816588

[65] Association AD. Standards of medical care in diabetes. Diabetes Care. 2014;**37**(Suppl 1):S14-S80

[66] Eurich DT, Majumdar SR, McAlister FA, et al. Improved clinical outcomes associated with metformin in patients with diabetes and heart failure. Diabetes Care. 2005;**28**:2345-2351

[67] Holman RR, Paul SK, Bethel MA, et al. 10-year follow-up of intensive glucose control in type 2 diabetes. The New England Journal of Medicine. 2008;**359**:1577-1589

[68] Pandey A, Kumar VL. Protective effect of metformin against acute inflammation and oxidative stress in rat. Drug Development Research. 2016;**77**:278-284

[69] Hattori Y, Hattori K, Hayashi T. Pleiotropic benefits of metformin: Macrophage targeting its anti-inflammatory mechanisms. Diabetes. 2015;**64**:1907-1909

[70] Iida KT, Kawakami Y, Suzuki M, et al. Effect of thiazolidinediones and metformin on LDL oxidation and aortic endothelium relaxation in diabetic GK rats. American Journal of Physiology. Endocrinology and Metabolism. 2003;**284**:E1125-E1130

[71] Rabbani N, Chittari MV, Bodmer CW, et al. Increased glycation and oxidative damage to apolipoprotein B100 of LDL cholesterol in patients with type 2 diabetes and effect of metformin. Diabetes. 2010;**59**:1038-1045

[72] Andersson C, Olesen JB, Hansen PR, et al. Metformin treatment is associated with a low risk of mortality in diabetic patients with heart failure: A retrospective nationwide cohort study. Diabetologia. 2010;**53**:2546-2553

[73] Aguilar D, Chan W, Bozkurt B, et al. Metformin use and mortality in ambulatory patients with diabetes and heart failure. Circulation. Heart Failure. 2011;**4**:53-58

[74] Lopaschuk GD. Metabolic abnormalities in the diabetic heart. Heart Failure Reviews. 2002;**7**:149-159

[75] Carroll R, Carley AN, Dyck JR, et al. Metabolic effects of insulin on cardiomyocytes from control and diabetic db/db mouse hearts. American Journal of Physiology. Endocrinology and Metabolism. 2005;**288**:E900-E906

[76] Buchanan J, Mazumder PK, Hu P, et al. Reduced cardiac efficiency and altered substrate metabolism precedes the onset of hyperglycemia and contractile dysfunction in two mouse models of insulin resistance and obesity. Endocrinology. 2005;**146**:5341-5349

[77] Sharma S, Adrogue JV, Golfman L, et al. Intramyocardial lipid accumulation in the failing human heart resembles the lipotoxic rat heart. The FASEB Journal. 2004;**18**:1692-1700

[78] Szczepaniak LS, Dobbins RL, Metzger GJ, et al. Myocardial triglycerides and systolic function in humans: in vivo evaluation by localized proton spectroscopy and cardiac imaging. Magnetic Resonance in Medicine. 2003;**49**:417-423

[79] Despres JP, Lemieux I. Abdominal obesity and metabolic syndrome. Nature. 2006;**444**:881-887

[80] Lewis GF, Carpentier A, Adeli K, et al. Disordered fat storage and mobilization in the pathogenesis of insulin resistance and type 2 diabetes. Endocrine Reviews. 2002;**23**:201-229

[81] Manzella D, Grella R, Esposito K, et al. Blood pressure and cardiac autonomic nervous system in obese type 2 diabetic patients: Effect of metformin administration. American Journal of Hypertension. 2004;**17**:223-227

[82] Jeppesen J, Zhou MY, Chen YD, et al. Effect of metformin on postprandial lipemia in patients with fairly to poorly controlled NIDDM. Diabetes Care. 1994;**17**:1093-1099

[83] Li J, Minczuk K, Massey JC, et al. Metformin improves cardiac metabolism and function, and prevents left ventricular hypertrophy in spontaneously hypertensive rats. Journal of the American Heart Association. 2020;**9**:e015154

[84] Yoon H, Cho HY, Yoo HD, et al. Influences of organic cation transporter polymorphisms on the population pharmacokinetics of metformin in healthy subjects. The AAPS Journal. 2013;**15**:571-580

[85] Falcao-Pires I, Leite-Moreira AF. Diabetic cardiomyopathy: Understanding the molecular and cellular basis to progress in diagnosis and treatment. Heart Failure Reviews. 2012;**17**:325-344

[86] Skrha J, Prazny M, Hilgertova J, et al. Oxidative stress and endothelium influenced by metformin in type 2 diabetes mellitus. European Journal of Clinical Pharmacology. 2007;**63**:1107-1114

[87] Beisswenger PJ, Howell SK, Touchette AD, et al. Metformin reduces systemic methylglyoxal levels in type 2 diabetes. Diabetes. 1999;**48**:198-202

[88] Scarpello JH, Howlett HC. Metformin therapy and clinical uses. Diabetes & Vascular Disease Research. 2008;**5**:157-167

[89] Ye G, Metreveli NS, Donthi RV, et al. Catalase protects cardiomyocyte function in models of type 1 and type 2 diabetes. Diabetes. 2004;**53**:1336-1343

[90] Shen X, Zheng S, Thongboonkerd V, et al. Cardiac mitochondrial damage and biogenesis in a chronic model of type 1 diabetes. American Journal of Physiology. Endocrinology and Metabolism. 2004;**287**:E896-E905

[91] Boudina S, Sena S, O'Neill BT, et al. Reduced mitochondrial oxidative capacity and increased mitochondrial uncoupling impair myocardial energetics in obesity. Circulation. 2005;**112**:2686-2695

[92] Anderson EJ, Kypson AP, Rodriguez E, et al. Substrate-specific derangements in mitochondrial metabolism and redox balance in the atrium of the type 2 diabetic human heart. Journal of the American College of Cardiology. 2009;**54**:1891-1898

[93] Bourassa MG, Gurné O, Bangdiwala SI, et al. Natural history and patterns of current practice in heart failure. Journal of the American College of Cardiology. 1993;**22**:A14-A19

[94] Investigators S, Yusuf S, Pitt B, et al. Effect of enalapril on survival in patients with reduced left ventricular ejection fractions and congestive heart failure. The New England Journal of Medicine. 1991;**325**:293-302

[95] Liu XD, Li YG, Wang GY, et al. Metformin protects high glucosecultured cardiomyocytes from oxidative stress by promoting NDUFA13 expression and mitochondrial biogenesis via the AMPK signaling pathway. Molecular Medicine Reports. 2020;**22**:5262-5270

[96] Wold LE, Ren J. Streptozotocin directly impairs cardiac contractile function in isolated ventricular myocytes via a p38 map kinase-dependent oxidative stress mechanism. Biochemical and Biophysical Research Communications. 2004;**318**:1066-1071

[97] Steinberg HO, Paradisi G, Hook G, et al. Free fatty acid elevation impairs insulin-mediated vasodilation and nitric oxide production. Diabetes. 2000;**49**:1231-1238

[98] Imrie H, Abbas A, Kearney M. Insulin resistance, lipotoxicity and endothelial dysfunction. Biochimica et Biophysica Acta. 2010;**1801**:320-326

[99] King MK, Coker ML, Goldberg A, et al. Selective matrix metalloproteinase inhibition with developing heart failure: Effects on left ventricular function and structure. Circulation Research. 2003;**92**:177-185

[100] Cesselli D, Jakoniuk I, Barlucchi L, et al. Oxidative stress-mediated cardiac cell death is a major determinant of ventricular dysfunction and failure in dog dilated cardiomyopathy. Circulation Research. 2001;**89**:279-286

[101] Ren XM, Zuo GF, Wu W, et al. Atorvastatin alleviates experimental diabetic cardiomyopathy by regulating the GSK-3beta-PP2Ac-NF-kappaB Signaling Axis. PLoS One. 2016;**11**:e0166740

[102] Cheng G, Li L. High-glucose-induced apoptosis, ROS production and pro-inflammatory response in cardiomyocytes is attenuated by metformin treatment via PP2A activation. Journal of Biosciences. 2020:45

[103] Rosen P, Wiernsperger NF. Metformin delays the manifestation of diabetes and vascular dysfunction in Goto-Kakizaki rats by reduction of mitochondrial oxidative stress. Diabetes/Metabolism Research and Reviews. 2006;**22**:323-330

[104] Pierce GN, Russell JC. Regulation of intracellular Ca2+ in the heart during diabetes. Cardiovascular Research. 1997;**34**:41-47

[105] Teshima Y, Takahashi N, Saikawa T, et al. Diminished expression of sarcoplasmic reticulum

Ca(2+)-ATPase and ryanodine sensitive Ca(2+)channel mRNA in streptozotocin-induced diabetic rat heart. Journal of Molecular and Cellular Cardiology. 2000;**32**:655-664

[106] Jweied EE, McKinney RD, Walker LA, et al. Depressed cardiac myofilament function in human diabetes mellitus. American Journal of Physiology. Heart and Circulatory Physiology. 2005;**289**:H2478-H2483

[107] Tang WH, Cheng WT, Kravtsov GM, et al. Cardiac contractile dysfunction during acute hyperglycemia due to impairment of SERCA by polyol pathway-mediated oxidative stress. American Journal of Physiology. Cell Physiology. 2010;**299**:C643-C653

[108] Zhang L, Cannell MB, Phillips AR, et al. Altered calcium homeostasis does not explain the contractile deficit of diabetic cardiomyopathy. Diabetes. 2008;**57**:2158-2166

[109] Angebault C, Panel M, Lacote M, et al. Metformin reverses the enhanced myocardial SR/ER-mitochondria interaction and impaired Complex I-driven respiration in dystrophin-deficient mice. Frontier in Cell Development Biology. 2020;**8**:609493

[110] Top WMC, Kooy A, Stehouwer CDA. Metformin: A narrative review of its potential benefits for cardiovascular disease, Cancer and dementia. Pharmaceuticals (Basel). 2022:15

[111] Roussel R, Travert F, Pasquet B, et al. Metformin use and mortality among patients with diabetes and atherothrombosis. Archives of Internal Medicine. 2010;**170**:1892-1899

[112] Pladevall M, Riera-Guardia N, Margulis AV, et al. Cardiovascular risk associated with the use of glitazones, metformin and sufonylureas: meta-analysis of published observational studies. BMC Cardiovascular Disorders. 2016;**16**:14

[113] Solskov L, Lofgren B, Kristiansen SB, et al. Metformin induces cardioprotection against ischaemia/reperfusion injury in the rat heart 24 hours after administration. Basic & Clinical Pharmacology & Toxicology. 2008;**103**:82-87

[114] El Messaoudi S, Rongen GA, Riksen NP. Metformin therapy in diabetes: The role of cardioprotection. Current Atherosclerosis Reports. 2013;**15**:314

[115] El Messaoudi S, Rongen GA, de Boer RA, et al. The cardioprotective effects of metformin. Current Opinion in Lipidology. 2011;**22**:445-453

[116] V, C., B. F, M. S et al. Reduction of myocardial infarct size by metformin in rats submitted to permanent left coronary artery ligation. Diabetes & Metabolism. 1988;**14**:591-595

[117] Calvert JW, Gundewar S, Jha S, et al. Acute metformin therapy confers cardioprotection against myocardial infarction via AMPK-eNOS-mediated signaling. Diabetes. 2008;**57**:696-705

[118] Legtenberg RJ, Houston RJ, Oeseburg B, et al. Metformin improves cardiac functional recovery after ischemia in rats. Hormone and Metabolic Research. 2002;**34**:182-185

[119] Paiva MA, Goncalves LM, Providencia LA, et al. Transitory activation of AMPK at reperfusion protects the ischaemic-reperfused rat myocardium against infarction. Cardiovascular Drugs and Therapy. 2010;**24**:25-32

[120] Hausenloy D. Inhibiting mitochondrial permeability transition pore opening: A new paradigm for myocardial preconditioning? Cardiovascular Research. 2002;**55**:534-543

[121] Cadenas S. ROS and redox signaling in myocardial ischemia-reperfusion injury and cardioprotection. Free Radical Biology & Medicine. 2018;**117**:76-89

[122] Bhamra GS, Hausenloy DJ, Davidson SM, et al. Metformin protects the ischemic heart by the Akt-mediated inhibition of mitochondrial permeability transition pore opening. Basic Research in Cardiology. 2008;**103**:274-284

[123] Kulaczkowska ZM, Wrobel M, Rokicka D, et al. Metformin in patients with type 2 diabetes mellitus and heart failure: A review. Endokrynologia Polska. 2021;**72**:163-170

[124] Yang F, Qin Y, Wang Y, et al. Metformin inhibits the NLRP3 inflammasome via AMPK/mTOR-dependent effects in diabetic cardiomyopathy. International Journal of Biological Sciences. 2019;**15**:1010-1019

[125] Lai YC, Tabima DM, Dube JJ, et al. SIRT3-AMP-activated protein kinase activation by nitrite and metformin improves Hyperglycemia and normalizes pulmonary hypertension associated with heart failure with preserved ejection fraction. Circulation. 2016;**133**:717-731

Section 3

Metformin: Therapeutic Applications Among No-Diabetic Patients

Chapter 4

Glycemic and Extraglycemic Effects of Metformin in Patients with Diabetes

Dario Rahelić and Zrinka Šakić

Abstract

For several decades, metformin has been the mainstay of treatment of type 2 diabetes (T2D), not only due to its remarkable efficacy in both monotherapy and combination therapy regimens, but also due to its favorable safety profile, weight neutrality, and low cost. Other advantages have been reported, including improvements in lipid profile and inflammatory markers and reports of cardioprotective effects, albeit with scant evidence. The modification of the cellular energy metabolism is the core of metformin's mode of action. Metformin works to lower serum glucose concentration by inhibiting hepatic gluconeogenesis and countering the action of glucagon. Secondarily, it enhances glucose uptake in peripheral tissues, predominantly in the muscles. Long-term and widespread use of metformin has shed light on its other potential uses mediated by its effects on deranged metabolic pathways. Moreover, metformin is gaining research interest by demonstrating its potential in the treatment of multiple disorders other than diabetes and has been proven to have anti-cancer, immunoregulatory, and anti-aging properties. As a result, metformin is currently being researched as a potential treatment option for various diseases.

Keywords: metformin, diabetes, extraglycemic effects, longevity, microbiome, anticancer

1. Introduction

Metformin is a widely utilized oral treatment for type 2 diabetes (T2D), FDA-approved since 1998, this guanidine derivative has been thoroughly researched in molecular, biochemical, animal, human, and epidemiological trials first for its glycemic effects, with additional effects noted later. Metformin has come under the spotlight for its pleiotropic effects, which include anti-inflammatory, immunomodulatory, antibacterial, antiviral, anticancer, anti-aging, hormone regulatory, cardioprotective, and anti-lipid effects [1, 2]. These vast effects have led to research showing shared molecular mechanisms and multiple effects on cellular, biochemical, and other signaling pathways in the body, resulting in complex positive effects, particularly during chronic use. Furthermore, these extra glycemic effects are potentiated by the treatment of T2D, a risk factor for many conditions, including cardiovascular disease, cancer, infections, and obesity. Its low side-effect risk, low cost, and widespread use

IntechOpen

strengthen the interest in using metformin for treating conditions other than T2D, with some researchers labeling it "the Aspirin of the twenty-first century."

2. Glycemic effects of metformin

In use for over 30 years, metformin is the most commonly prescribed oral antihyperglycemic and is the first-line treatment for T2D. It acts primarily by decreasing hepatic glucose production, with additional effects by decreasing intestinal absorption of glucose and improving peripheral glucose uptake (**Figure 1**). Hypoglycemia is unlikely with metformin, making its side effects more favorable when compared to other, older oral antihyperglycemics such as sulfonylureas. In primary hepatocytes, metformin activates the AMP-activated protein kinase (AMPK) pathway, which results in the inhibition of glucose production [3, 4]. Additionally, recent advances have shown that metformin's effects on gluconeogenesis may be independent of AMPK activation. Metformin acts on the respiratory chain in mitochondria, changing the intracellular ATP levels, thereby impairing the supply of ATP required for gluconeogenesis [3–6]. Another recently reported potential target of metformin may be mitochondrial glycerophosphate dehydrogenase [7]. Other mechanisms of metformin on glycemia include potential improvements in homeostasis *via* actions on glucagon-like peptide 1 and antagonization of glucagon, further suppressing hepatic gluconeogenesis [8–10].

The effect of metformin on the intestines involves several mechanisms. Fundamentally, metformin decreases proximal intestinal glucose absorption, possibly by increasing enterocytic glucose utilization and increased lactate production [11].

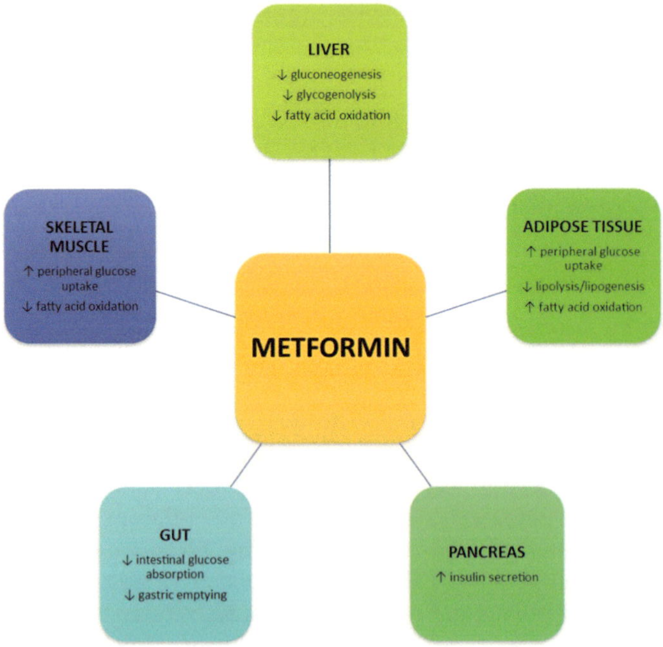

Figure 1.
Overview of metformin glycemic effects.

The complete mechanisms by which glucose utilization is increased are unclear; however, animal models indicate a role in increased GLUT2 expression on the enterocyte membrane. The other pathways of metformin's action on the gut involve its effects on the incretin system. Metformin increases GLP-1 secretion by enteroendocrine cells in the intestine, thereby enhancing glucose homeostasis. Mechanisms of this GLP-1 increase are under debate, and the currently prevailing opinion is that metformin acts by increasing GLP-1 production rather than by preventing its degradation by DPP-4 [12, 13]. Other glucoregulatory effects *via* the intestines include modulations of the gut-brain axis and its effects on the intestinal microbiome [14].

Metformin reduces gluconeogenesis and hepatic glucose production, increasing peripheral glucose uptake and improving insulin sensitivity.

3. Extraglycemic effects of metformin

3.1 Metformin and aging

Aging is an inevitable biological process occurring in all organisms and is defined by the accumulation of numerous detrimental alterations that are correlated with an increased risk for morbidity and mortality. Although aging itself cannot be called a disease, it is undeniable that age-related disorders are one of the major causes of mortality worldwide. Aging is regulated by numerous cellular signaling mechanisms, namely protein homeostasis, nutrient-sensing pathways, and ROS-mediated oxidative stress [15]. In recent years, there has been considerable interest in researching metformin as an anti-aging medicine that could not only improve health but also increase lifespan. Research showed that metformin can increase lifespan by modulating the generation of ROS *via* the SIRT-3, Nrf-2/GPx7, and PRDX-2/SKN-1 signaling pathways [16–18]. Furthermore, it was established that it promotes the autophagy-mediated clearance of decaying components while reducing mTOR-induced production of aging-related proteins (e.g., progerin). Several studies have already demonstrated metformin's positive effect on aging in humans. Metformin in longevity study (MILES) is a 3-year trial in which 14 senior individuals with impaired glucose tolerance were treated with metformin at 1700 mg/day. The findings of the study showed that metformin administration caused transcriptome alterations in aging-related pathways, such as mitochondrial pathways, adipose tissue, fatty acid metabolism, and DNA repair processes [19]. Campbell et al. conducted a systematic review and a meta-analysis of 53 studies that showed that metformin might enhance both health span and longevity irrespective of its antihyperglycemic effects, implying that metformin fits the criteria for the anti-aging medication [20]. Likewise, an analysis of over 180,000 T2D patients' medical records from the UK Clinical Practice Research Datalink indicated that, despite being more obese and having more comorbidities than their non-diabetic counterparts, metformin-treated diabetic patients had survival rates comparable to their matched nondiabetic control group [21]. On the other hand, some studies demonstrated that metformin is less effective than exercise and may negate some of the benefits of exercise [22, 23]. Despite mentioned positive findings, metformin should be used with caution beyond the treatment of T2D, particularly in older people who may be at risk of metformin toxicity due to their possible hepatic and renal impairment. Further research is needed to demonstrate metformin as potential prophylaxis for age-related complications.

3.2 Metformin and cancer

Diabetes types 1 and 2 are both associated with increased rates of developing certain types of cancer, a link noticed over 90 years ago [24]. Common risk factors for diabetes and certain cancer types deepen the correlation among these entities. Bearing this in mind, could treatment or prevention of diabetes play a role in cancer incidence? This large and productive study question was initiated by a 2005 epidemiological report describing a link between metformin use and decreased rates of cancer occurrence [25]. Similar observational studies of patients with diabetes type 2 with or without metformin report lower cancer incidence in patients on metformin [26]. This sparked numerous *in-vitro*, animal, retrospective, prospective, and randomized controlled trials (RCTs), with several hundred registered RCTs investigating the effects of metformin on different cancer types currently in progress. *In-vitro* and animal studies have shown elaborate evidence of the anticancer effects of metformin as well as its modes of action on various mechanisms in cancer cells. Metformin has been shown to disrupt cellular energy mechanisms by affecting AMPK and mTOR pathways and by decreasing available glucose, has further effects on inhibition of protein synthesis and cell growth, as well as anti-angiogenic and anti-inflammatory effects [2, 27]. An important barrier to translating the findings of *in-vitro* and animal studies is the concentration of metformin used to achieve these effects, which is frequently 10–1000x times higher than the usual human dose. However, after oral intake, metformin distribution is different across the body, and for certain targets, such as the gastrointestinal, hepatic, and urinary systems, reaching these concentrations is possible. In the gut, the concentration of metformin remains 30–300 times higher than in plasma. At the same time, imaging studies show metformin accumulates in the liver, kidneys, and urinary bladder at concentrations far higher than those in plasma [28–30]. Another important factor for the responsiveness of cells was the expression of organic cation transporters, whose increased expression enables a very high concentration of metformin in the endoplasmic reticulum and mitochondria [31]. A wide body of findings indicates a potentially high therapeutic potential of metformin in cancer, particularly in these organ systems. However, definitive evidence of its beneficial effects, particularly in human studies, is lacking and often contradicting. It is studied for various cancer types at various stages, such as prevention, chemotherapeutic and neoadjuvant treatment. Meta-analysis of observational studies showed a 31% overall relative risk reduction (CI 0.61–0.79) for overall cancer development in participants taking metformin compared with other antidiabetic drugs. Promising trends were noted for breast, colon, pancreatic, and hepatocellular cancer [32]. Epidemiological and observational studies show a risk reduction of colorectal cancer incidence in metformin users, particularly diabetics. However, no RCTs have identified any association, but a protective effect was noted when metformin was compared to other antihyperglycemics [33, 34]. Similarly, for pancreatic cancer, observational and epidemiological studies show a 44% risk reduction, while RCTs show no protective effects of metformin. A systematic review of an RCT and nine observational studies for liver cancer showed a significant protective effect (OR 0.34; CI 0.19–0.60). As for pancreatic and colorectal cancer, observational studies showed a protective effect on stomach cancer, however, when pooled with results from RCTs, the protective effect was lost. Melanoma, prostate, kidney, lung, ovarian, and uterine cancer all showed no beneficial effects from metformin in both observational studies and RCTs, albeit metformin had a marginally protective effect against lung cancer in observational studies [34]. Its lack of effect on advanced cancer independent of the site or type of cancer was demonstrated in a recent meta-analysis [35].

Overall, the vast heterogeneity of published data indicates the need for meticulous RCTs with long follow-ups and adequate confounder control to fully investigate metformin's anticancer effects in humans for prevention, chemotherapy, or neoadjuvant treatment. Several hundred registered ongoing RCTs promise to elucidate the potential of metformin in cancer treatment.

3.3 Metformin and gut microbiota

Numerous microorganisms have a critical role in physiologic and metabolic processes in our body. Their habitat is mainly in our gut and therefore are called "gut flora" or "gut microbiota." The composition of the microbiota is influenced by both internal and external factors, such as the type of delivery, nutrition, exposure to antibiotics, gut inflammation, stress, menopause, and toxins. The process of altering the predominant microbiota is known as dysbiosis, and it has been linked to the development of various illnesses. The internal gut medium can be aggrieved by changes in the microbiome in a variety of ways, including altered pancreatic enzyme function, biliary acid degradation, damage to the intestinal brush border, and the development of dysregulated immunological responses due to bacterial antigens. These changes, however, are reversible [36]. There is a strong correlation between the incidence of inflammatory diseases and disturbance in the microbiome composition. The gut microbiota interacts closely with the inflammatory, renal, cardiovascular, and endocrine systems *via* metabolic, humoral, and neural signaling pathways [37]. Several important molecular and pathophysiologic mechanisms linking the microbiome, obesity, and diabetes mellitus have been elucidated, most prominently low grade-inflammation, lipopolysaccharides, bile acids, short-chain fatty acids (SCFAs), and reduced intestinal permeability [38]. Of note, besides their direct effects on glucose homeostasis and insulin resistance, the effects of intestinal microbiota span to other factors in diabetes development, like body mass index (BMI) and low-grade inflammation, as well as the consequences of existing DM, including chronic kidney disease and diabetic retinopathy [37].

Novel studies have shown the effects of metformin on the composition of the gut microbiome, resulting in changes affecting several processes and diseases, including effects on diabetes mellitus, the cardiovascular system, and aging (**Figure 2**) [39]. The half-life of metformin in the blood is 3–4 hours, while its glucose-lowering effects are observed for much longer. Furthermore, glucose lowering was shown to be stronger after intraduodenal than intravenous administration [13, 39]. Metformin treatment has been shown to result in positive changes in the microbiome composition both in animal models and humans, namely, increased relative rates of *Akkermansia* and *Firmicutes*/*Bacteroides* ratio [13, 40]. Even short-term metformin treatment is associated with a lowered abundance of *Bacteroides fragilis* in the intestine, leading to improved glucose tolerance, which was reversed when *B. fragilis* was reintroduced to the gut [41]. A randomized double-blind trial investigated the treatment of naïve T2DM patients versus placebo and showed improved glucose tolerance in mice with fecal transplants from metformin-treated patients. This indicated that the glucose-lowering effect of metformin is at least partially mediated by its effect on the microbiome [42]. The study conducted by Zhang et al. concluded that metformin modulated gut microbiota and contributed to the increase of SCFA metabolizing bacteria in treated rats [43].

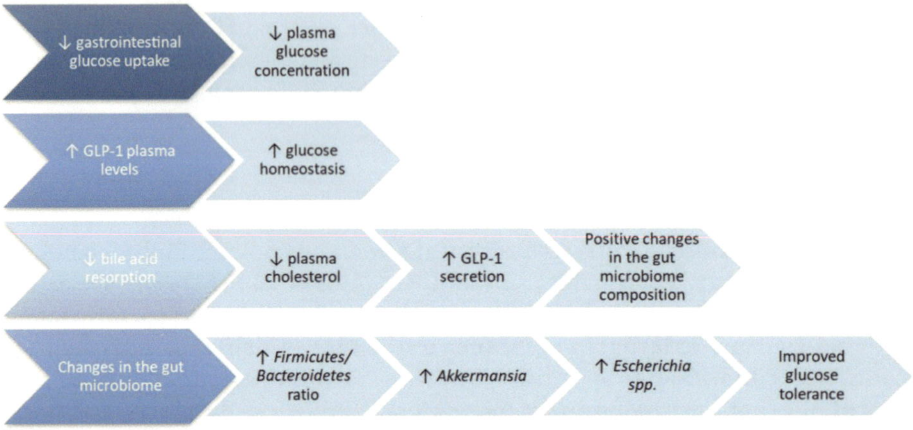

Figure 2.
Effects of metformin on diabetes via the gastrointestinal tract.

Metformin affects glycemia *via* several mechanisms resulting in a decrease of intestinal glucose absorption, positive changes in the gut microbiome leading to decreased "intestinal leak" and lower circulatory levels of proinflammatory cytokines resulting in improved glucose homeostasis. Decreased bile acid resorption has positive effects on the plasma lipid profile, as well as additional effects on glucose homeostasis *via* increased glucagon-like peptide 1 (GLP-1) secretion and changes associated with positive alterations of the intestinal microbiome.

3.4 Other extraglycemic effects of metformin

3.4.1 Polycystic ovary syndrome

Polycystic ovary syndrome (PCOS) is an endocrine disorder marked by hyperandrogenism, polycystic ovaries, and disorders of ovulation, making it one of the most common causes of female infertility. It is a heterogeneous condition also associated with features of metabolic syndrome. Prevalence of PCOS, based on the Rotterdam consensus workshop, rates up to 15% [44]. Insulin resistance in women with PCOS was first described by Burghen et al. in 1980 [45]. Weight gain is associated with insulin resistance in both women with and without PCOS; however, PCOS is associated with insulin resistance even in 75% of lean women with PCOS, albeit less severe than in obese women with PCOS [46]. Another important component of metabolic derangements in PCOS is dyslipidemia, most commonly manifested as increased LDL and total cholesterol [47]. Interestingly, genes most commonly associated with PCOS are genes related to the insulin receptor, primarily insulin receptor substrate 1 and 2 (IRS-1 and 2), calpain 10, genes for the expression of androgen-producing enzymes, and polymorphisms peroxisome proliferator-activated receptor gamma (PPARγ) [48]. These findings represent the basis for the use of "insulin-sensitizers," such as metformin, for the treatment of PCOS. Studies show that the combination of metformin and lifestyle changes leads to more weight loss and improved menstrual cycle regularity when compared to lifestyle changes alone. The proposed benefits of metformin in PCOS stem from its effects on weight loss, lowering of serum testosterone, and beneficial effects on dyslipidemia and endothelial function [49]. Metformin improves menstrual regularity, an effect more pronounced in lean patients, even those who are underweight [50]. Women (particularly obese) with PCOS are significantly more insulin resistant than their age- and BMI-matched female counterparts. Adipose tissue deposition in women with PCOS is more pronounced in the visceral and abdominal areas, termed android body fat distribution. Such fat deposition has adverse effects on hyperinsulinemia, causing consequent co-gonadotropic effects on the ovaries. Additionally, it endorses further android fat generation exacerbating weight gain [51]. Metformin does not primarily target fat tissue. Moreover, its effects on adipose tissue are unclear and many findings are debated. Many *in-vitro* and animal findings, such as increased glucose uptake and metabolism by adipocytes, effects on mitochondrial and peroxisomal fatty acid oxidation, lipolysis, and aerobic and anaerobic respiration, are yet unproven in human studies [49]. However, metformin may affect adipocytes through the activation of AMPK, which results in counteraction to the obesogenic effects of corticosteroids [52]. Metformin reduces hyperinsulinemia, effectively and safely ameliorating the reproductive, metabolic, and cardiovascular morbidity in PCOS. Metformin seems to have additional effects on the ovary itself. All current studies are *in-vitro* studies, and the exact mode of action is unclear. So far, it appears that metformin inhibits androgen production in human ovarian granulosa cells [53]. Metformin is a drug for all reasons. Other observed modes of action include AMPK-related pathways, similar to those in other tissues. In rat granulosa cells, metformin treatment resulted in AMPK activation and reduced steroidogenesis [54]. Studies evaluating pregnancy outcomes in women with PCOS remain inconclusive. In some patients, improved pregnancy outcomes could be a result of attenuation of hyperinsulinemia, reduced insulin resistance, and inhibition of the plasminogen activator, resulting in improved oocyte quality and folliculogenesis [55]. However, due to the non-significant improvement in outcomes, the use of metformin only in patients with impaired glucose tolerance [56].

3.4.2 Non-alcoholic fatty liver disease

Non-alcoholic fatty liver disease (NAFLD) is a term used for liver disorders often seen in obese individuals, particularly those with type 2 diabetes. These disorders include simple fatty liver disease, non-alcoholic steatohepatitis (NASH), liver fibrosis, cirrhosis, and hepatocellular carcinoma (HCC). The prevalence of NAFLD in people with diabetes is between 50 and 90% [57]. Because of this high correlation, NAFLD is considered a novel T2D predictive indicator [58]. Initial treatment of NAFLD, as well as diabetes, includes weight loss and lifestyle changes to improve insulin sensitivity, reduce serum liver enzyme levels, and lower the degree of fatty change in the liver. Metformin has been shown to suppress hepatic gluconeogenesis, change hepatic fatty acid metabolism, increase fatty acid oxidation, suppress lipogenesis, and improve insulin sensitivity. Recently, it was revealed that metformin has beneficial effects on liver histology in patients with NAFLD/NASH [59]. Nonetheless, metformin is commonly prescribed off-label to patients with NAFLD since it is thought that activation of AMPK is associated with a myriad of positive benefits, such as reduction in oxidative stress and liver inflammation [60]. However, its long-term clinical effects on NASH patients, particularly in lowering the risk of HCC in NAFLD/NASH patients, are unknown. Patients with established T2D should be evaluated for NAFLD as it contributes to the progression of diabetes (**Figure 3**). Because viable noninvasive diagnostics for histological and biochemical indicators of NASH are unavailable, liver biopsy remains the current gold standard for diagnosis. The most practical approach

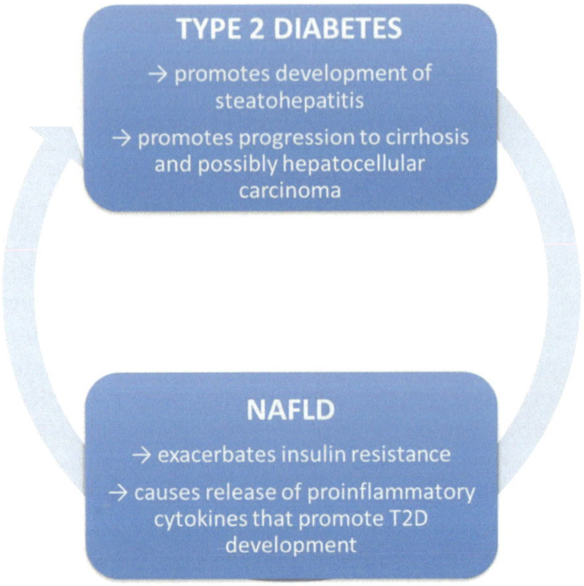

Figure 3.
Relationship between type 2 diabetes (T2D) and non-alcoholic fatty liver disease (NAFLD).

for detecting NAFLD is liver ultrasonography; however, it has yet to be proven for monitoring response to treatment. Therefore, metabolic markers remain viable indicators of therapeutic response.

In NAFLD the lipid accumulation within hepatocytes results in hepatic insulin resistance, hepatic insulin clearance is reduced and toxic cytokines are released which promotes the development of T2D. Type 2 diabetes is associated with higher rates of development of steatohepatitis, progression to liver cirrhosis, and possibly the development of hepatocellular carcinoma.

4. Future perspective

The described pleiotropic effects of metformin may be potentiated or affected when used in combination with other oral antihyperglycemic drugs. Frequently, the choice of second-agent drugs is dependent on the comorbidities, cost, and target goals individually tailored for each patient. The combined effects of other drugs, including GLP-1 receptor agonists, SGLT2 inhibitors, and DPP-4 are the focus of current research investigating their combined effects on glycemic control as well as influences outside regulation of plasma glucose concentration. In light of the new evidence and effects of other oral antihyperglycemics on the cardiovascular and renal systems, the Japanese guidelines are the first not to recommend metformin as a first-choice agent, but rather, one of the possible choices for first-line monotherapy. Other guidelines, including Korean and the American Diabetes Associations, recommend including different oral antihyperglycemics earlier than before [61]. Combination therapy of metformin with additional one or two drugs is currently being investigated for long-term safety and glycemic control. A recent study compared a metformin-DPP4 inhibitor combination compared to metformin, DPP-4, and an SGLT2 inhibitor, and the results showed similar long-term glycemic control, indicating better cost-effectiveness of dual than triple therapy [62]. Of note, extraglycemic effects were more pronounced in patients on triple therapy; however, in selected populations, dual therapy may be similarly effective at a lower cost. Long-term efficacy studies and cost-effectiveness need to be studied for all possible combinations, and the results of these studies may guide physicians in selecting more appropriate treatments for their patients.

5. Conclusion

Metformin has been the first-line treatment for T2D for decades. The advantages of using metformin include its safety profile and low cost compared to newer medications such as GLP-1 receptor agonists and SGLT-2 inhibitors. Apart from its usage in the treatment of diabetes, growing evidence suggests that metformin may be beneficial in the treatment of cancer, PCOS, NAFLD, and a variety of other chronic diseases. By its effects on glucose homeostasis, the incretin axis, lipid metabolism, and the gut microbiome, it is reasonable to assume that metformin has a multitude of roles in disorders other than diabetes, and consequently, may increase healthspan and longevity.

Conflict of interest

The authors declare no conflict of interest.

Author details

Dario Rahelić[1,2]* and Zrinka Šakić[1]

1 Vuk Vrhovac University Clinic for Diabetes, Endocrinology and Metabolic Diseases, Merkur University Hospital, Zagreb, Croatia

2 Catholic University of Croatia School of Medicine, Zagreb, Croatia

*Address all correspondence to: dario.rahelic@gmail.com

References

[1] Ursini F, Russo E, Pellino G, D'Angelo S, Chiaravalloti A, De Sarro G, et al. Metformin and autoimmunity: A "new deal" of an old drug. Frontiers in Immunology. 2018;**9**:1236

[2] Triggle CR, Mohammed I, Bshesh K, Marei I, Ye K, Ding H, et al. Metformin: Is it a drug for all reasons and diseases? Metabolism. 2022;**133**:155223

[3] Foretz M, Guigas B, Bertrand L, Pollak M, Viollet B. Metformin: From mechanisms of action to therapies. Cell Metabolism. 2014;**20**(6):953-966

[4] Miller RA, Chu Q, Xie J, Foretz M, Viollet B, Birnbaum MJ. Biguanides suppress hepatic glucagon signaling by decreasing the production of cyclic AMP. Nature. 2013;**494**(7436):256-260

[5] Hawley SA, Ross FA, Chevtzoff C, Green KA, Evans A, Fogarty S, et al. Use of cells expressing gamma subunit variants to identify diverse mechanisms of AMPK activation. Cell Metabolism. 2010;**11**(6):554-565

[6] Foretz M, Hébrard S, Leclerc J, Zarrinpashneh E, Soty M, Mithieux G, et al. Metformin inhibits hepatic gluconeogenesis in mice independently of the LKB1/AMPK pathway via a decrease in hepatic energy state. The Journal of Clinical Investigation. 2010;**120**(7):2355-2369

[7] Madiraju AK, Erion DM, Rahimi Y, Zhang X-M, Braddock DT, Albright RA, et al. Metformin suppresses gluconeogenesis by inhibiting mitochondrial glycerophosphate dehydrogenase. Nature. 2014;**510**(7506):542-546

[8] Maida A, Lamont BJ, Cao X, Drucker DJ. Metformin regulates the incretin receptor axis via a pathway dependent on peroxisome proliferator-activated receptor-α in mice. Diabetologia. 2011;**54**(2):339-349

[9] Mulherin AJ, Oh AH, Kim H, Grieco A, Lauffer LM, Brubaker PL. Mechanisms underlying metformin-induced secretion of glucagon-like peptide-1 from the intestinal L cell. Endocrinology. 2011;**152**(12):4610-4619

[10] Cuthbertson J, Patterson S, O'Harte FP, Bell PM. Addition of metformin to exogenous glucagon-like peptide-1 results in increased serum glucagon-like peptide-1 concentrations and greater glucose lowering in type 2 diabetes mellitus. Metabolism. 2011;**60**(1):52-56

[11] Bailey CJ, Mynett KJ, Page T. Importance of the intestine as a site of metformin-stimulated glucose utilization. British Journal of Pharmacology. 1994;**112**(2):671-675

[12] McCreight LJ, Bailey CJ, Pearson ER. Metformin and the gastrointestinal tract. Diabetologia. 2016;**59**(3):426-435

[13] Wu T, Horowitz M, Rayner CK. New insights into the anti-diabetic actions of metformin: From the liver to the gut. Expert Review of Gastroenterology & Hepatology. 2017;**11**(2):157-166

[14] Foretz M, Guigas B, Viollet B. Understanding the glucoregulatory mechanisms of metformin in type 2 diabetes mellitus. Nature Reviews. Endocrinology. 2019;**15**(10):569-589

[15] Hsu S-K, Cheng K-C, Mgbeahuruike MO, Lin Y-H, Wu C-Y, Wang H-MD, et al. New insight into the effects of metformin on

diabetic retinopathy, aging and cancer: Nonapoptotic cell death, immunosuppression, and effects beyond the AMPK pathway. International Journal of Molecular Sciences. 2021;**22**(17):9453. [Published: 31 August 2021]

[16] De Haes W, Frooninckx L, Van Assche R, Smolders A, Depuydt G, Billen J, et al. Metformin promotes lifespan through mitohormesis via the peroxiredoxin PRDX-2. Proceedings of the National Academy of Sciences of the United States of America. 2014;**111**(24):E2501-E2509

[17] Fang J, Yang J, Wu X, Zhang G, Li T, Wang X, et al. Metformin alleviates human cellular aging by upregulating the endoplasmic reticulum glutathione peroxidase 7. Aging Cell. 2018;**17**(4):e12765

[18] Karnewar S, Neeli PK, Panuganti D, Kotagiri S, Mallappa S, Jain N, et al. Metformin regulates mitochondrial biogenesis and senescence through AMPK mediated H3K79 methylation: Relevance in age-associated vascular dysfunction. Biochimica et Biophysica Acta - Molecular Basis of Disease. 2018;**1864**(4 Pt A):1115-1128

[19] Kulkarni AS, Brutsaert EF, Anghel V, Zhang K, Bloomgarden N, Pollak M, et al. Metformin regulates metabolic and nonmetabolic pathways in skeletal muscle and subcutaneous adipose tissues of older adults. Aging Cell. 2018;**17**(2):e12723

[20] Campbell JM, Bellman SM, Stephenson MD, Lisy K. Metformin reduces all-cause mortality and diseases of aging independent of its effect on diabetes control: A systematic review and meta-analysis. Ageing Research Reviews. 2017;**40**:31-44

[21] Bannister CA, Holden SE, Jenkins-Jones S, Morgan CL, Halcox JP, Schernthaner G, et al. Can people with type 2 diabetes live longer than those without? A comparison of mortality in people initiated with metformin or sulphonylurea monotherapy and matched non-diabetic controls. Diabetes, Obesity & Metabolism. 2014;**16**(11):1165-1173

[22] Malin SK, Braun B. Impact of metformin on exercise-induced metabolic adaptations to lower type 2 diabetes risk. Exercise and Sport Sciences Reviews. Jan 2016;**44**(1):4-11

[23] Konopka AR, Laurin JL, Schoenberg HM, Reid JJ, Castor WM, Wolff CA, et al. Metformin inhibits mitochondrial adaptations to aerobic exercise training in older adults. Aging Cell. 2019;**18**(1):e12880

[24] Wilson EB, Maher HC. Cancer and tuberculosis with some comments on cancer and other diseases. American Journal of Cancer Research. 1932;**16**(2):227-250

[25] Evans JMM, Donnelly LA, Emslie-Smith AM, Alessi DR, Morris AD. Metformin and reduced risk of cancer in diabetic patients. BMJ. 2005;**330**(7503):1304-1305

[26] Kim HJ, Lee S, Chun KH, Jeon JY, Han SJ, Kim DJ, et al. Metformin reduces the risk of cancer in patients with type 2 diabetes: An analysis based on the Korean National Diabetes Program Cohort. Medicine (Baltimore). 2018;**97**(8):e0036

[27] Morale MG, Tamura RE, Rubio IGS. Metformin and cancer hallmarks: Molecular mechanisms in thyroid, prostate and head and neck cancer models. Biomolecules. 2022;**12**(3):357

[28] Bailey CJ, Wilcock C, Scarpello JHB. Metformin and the intestine. Diabetologia. 2008;**51**:1552-1553

[29] Gormsen LC, Sundelin EI, Jensen JB, Vendelbo MH, Jakobsen S, Munk OL, et al. In vivo imaging of human 11C-metformin in peripheral organs: Dosimetry, biodistribution, and kinetic analyses. Journal of Nuclear Medicine. 2016;**57**(12):1920-1926

[30] Marini C, Cossu V, Bauckneht M, Lanfranchi F, Raffa S, Orengo AM, et al. Metformin and cancer glucose metabolism: At the bench or at the bedside? Biomolecules. 2021;**11**(8):1231

[31] Chien H-C, Zur AA, Maurer TS, Yee SW, Tolsma J, Jasper P, et al. Rapid method to determine intracellular drug concentrations in cellular uptake assays: Application to metformin in organic cation transporter 1-transfected human embryonic kidney 293 cells. Drug Metabolism and Disposition. 2016;**44**(3):356-364

[32] DeCensi A, Puntoni M, Goodwin P, Cazzaniga M, Gennari A, Bonanni B, et al. Metformin and cancer risk in diabetic patients: A systematic review and meta-analysis. Cancer Prevention Research. 2010;**3**(11):1451-1461

[33] Lee M-S, Hsu C-C, Wahlqvist ML, Tsai H-N, Chang Y-H, Huang Y-C. Type 2 diabetes increases and metformin reduces total, colorectal, liver, and pancreatic cancer incidences in Taiwanese: A representative population prospective cohort study of 800,000 individuals. BMC Cancer. 2011;**11**:20

[34] Franciosi M, Lucisano G, Lapice E, Strippoli GFM, Pellegrini F, Nicolucci A. Metformin therapy and risk of cancer in patients with type 2 diabetes: Systematic review. PLoS One. 2013;**8**(8):e71583

[35] Gan X, Cao C, He Y, Hu X, Peng X, Su Y. Metformin has no significant anticancer effect on patients with advanced or unresectable cancer: A systematic review and meta-analysis. Current Pharmaceutical Design. 2022;**28**:1351-1358

[36] Carding S, Verbeke K, Vipond DT, Corfe BM, Owen LJ. Dysbiosis of the gut microbiota in disease. Microbial Ecology in Health and Disease. 2015;**26**:26191

[37] Kanbay M, Onal EM, Afsar B, Dagel T, Yerlikaya A, Covic A, et al. The crosstalk of gut microbiota and chronic kidney disease: Role of inflammation, proteinuria, hypertension, and diabetes mellitus. International Urology and Nephrology. 2018;**50**(8):1453-1466

[38] Singer-Englar T, Barlow G, Mathur R. Obesity, diabetes, and the gut microbiome: An updated review. Expert Review of Gastroenterology & Hepatology. 2019;**13**(1):3-15

[39] Pascale A, Marchesi N, Govoni S, Coppola A, Gazzaruso C. The role of gut microbiota in obesity, diabetes mellitus, and effect of metformin: New insights into old diseases. Current Opinion in Pharmacology. 2019;**49**:1-5

[40] Yerevanian A, Soukas AA. Metformin: Mechanisms in human obesity and weight loss. Current Obesity Reports. 2019;**8**(2):156-164

[41] Sun L, Xie C, Wang G, Wu Y, Wu Q, Wang X, et al. Gut microbiota and intestinal FXR mediate the clinical benefits of metformin. Nature Medicine. 2018;**24**(12):1919-1929

[42] Wu H, Esteve E, Tremaroli V, Khan MT, Caesar R, Mannerås-Holm L, et al. Metformin alters the gut microbiome of individuals with treatment-naive type 2 diabetes, contributing to the therapeutic effects of the drug. Nature Medicine. 2017;**23**(7):850-858

[43] Zhang X, Zhao Y, Xu J, Xue Z, Zhang M, Pang X, et al. Modulation of gut microbiota by berberine and metformin during the treatment of high-fat diet-induced obesity in rats. Scientific Reports. 2015;**5**:14405

[44] Rotterdam ESHRE/ASRM-Sponsored PCOS Consensus Workshop Group. Revised 2003 consensus on diagnostic criteria and long-term health risks related to polycystic ovary syndrome. Fertility and Sterility. 2004;**81**(1):19-25. DOI: 10.1016/j.fertnstert.2003.10.004

[45] Burghen GA, Givens JR, Kitabchi AE. Correlation of hyperandrogenism with hyperinsulinism in polycystic ovarian disease. The Journal of Clinical Endocrinology and Metabolism. 1980;**50**(1):113-116

[46] Stepto NK, Cassar S, Joham AE, Hutchison SK, Harrison CL, Goldstein RF, et al. Women with polycystic ovary syndrome have intrinsic insulin resistance on the euglycaemic–hyperinsulinemic clamp. Human Reproduction. 2013;**28**(3):777-784. DOI: 10.1093/humrep/des463

[47] Toosy S, Sodi R, Pappachan JM. Lean polycystic ovary syndrome (PCOS): An evidence-based practical approach. Journal of Diabetes and Metabolic Disorders. 2018;**17**(2):277-285

[48] Hardy OT, Czech MP, Corvera S. What causes the insulin resistance underlying obesity? Current Opinion in Endocrinology, Diabetes, and Obesity. 2012;**19**(2):81-87

[49] Diamanti-KandarakisE,ChristakouCD, Kandaraki E, Economou FN. Metformin: An old medication of new fashion: Evolving new molecular mechanisms and clinical implications in polycystic ovary syndrome. European Journal of Endocrinology. 2010;**162**(2):193-212

[50] Anastasiou OE, Canbay A, Fuhrer D, Reger-Tan S. Metabolic and androgen profile in underweight women with polycystic ovary syndrome. Archives of Gynecology and Obstetrics. 2017;**296**(2):363-371

[51] Barber TM, McCarthy MI, Wass JAH, Franks S. Obesity and polycystic ovary syndrome. Clinical Endocrinology. 2006;**65**(2):137-145

[52] Christ-Crain M, Kola B, Lolli F, Fekete C, Seboek D, Wittmann G, et al. AMP-activated protein kinase mediates glucocorticoid-induced metabolic changes: A novel mechanism in Cushing's syndrome. The FASEB Journal. 2008;**22**(6):1672-1683. DOI: 10.1096/fj.07-094144

[53] Mansfield R, Galea R, Brincat M, Hole D, Mason H. Metformin has direct effects on human ovarian steroidogenesis. Fertility and Sterility. 2003;**79**(4):956-962

[54] Tosca L, Solnais P, Ferré P, Foufelle F, Dupont J. Metformin-induced stimulation of adenosine 5′ monophosphate-activated protein kinase (PRKA) impairs progesterone secretion in rat granulosa cells. Biology of Reproduction. 2006;**75**(3):342-351. DOI: 10.1095/biolreprod.106.050831

[55] Glueck CJ, Streicher P, Wang P. Treatment of polycystic ovary syndrome with insulin-lowering agents. Expert Opinion on Pharmacotherapy. 2002;**3**(8):1177-1189

[56] Messinis IE, Messini CI, Anifandis G, Dafopoulos K. Polycystic ovaries and obesity. Best Practice & Research. Clinical Obstetrics & Gynaecology. 2015;**29**(4):479-488

[57] Chan W-K, Tan AT-B, Vethakkan SR, Tah P-C, Vijayananthan A, Goh K-L.

Non-alcoholic fatty liver disease in diabetics—Prevalence and predictive factors in a multiracial hospital clinic population in Malaysia. Journal of Gastroenterology and Hepatology. 2013;**28**(8):1375-1383

[58] Fruci B, Giuliano S, Mazza A, Malaguarnera R, Belfiore A. Nonalcoholic fatty liver: A possible new target for type 2 diabetes prevention and treatment. International Journal of Molecular Sciences. 2013;**14**(11):22933-22966

[59] Said A, Akhter A. Meta-analysis of randomized controlled trials of pharmacologic agents in non-alcoholic steatohepatitis. Annals of Hepatology. 2017;**16**(4):538-547

[60] Smith BK, Marcinko K, Desjardins EM, Lally JS, Ford RJ, Steinberg GR. Treatment of nonalcoholic fatty liver disease: Role of AMPK. American Journal of Physiology. Endocrinology and Metabolism. 2016;**311**(4):E730-E740

[61] Yu J, Lee SH, Kim MK. Recent updates to clinical practice guidelines for diabetes mellitus. Endocrinology and Metabolism. 2022;**37**(1):26-37. DOI: 10.3803/EnM.2022.105

[62] Lin YY, Weng SF, Hsu CH, et al. Effect of metformin monotherapy and dual or triple concomitant therapy with metformin on glycemic control and lipid profile management of patients with type 2 diabetes mellitus. Frontiers in Medicine. 2022;**9**:995944. DOI: 10.3389/fmed.2022.995944 [Published: 14 October 2022]

Chapter 5

Metformin in Non-Diabetic Conditions: An Overview

Shafaat Husain Talib, Umar Quadri, Sachin Patel and Pranita Barapatre

Abstract

Metformin has been proven to be one of the most safe and effective antihyperglycemic agent. Jean Sterne in 1957 first used metformin for treatment of diabetes mellitus type II. The main effect of this drug from the biguanide family is to acutely decrease hepatic glucose production, mostly through a mild and transient inhibition of the mitochondrial respiratory chain complex I. The drug is an insulin sensitizer, leading to reduction in insulin resistance and significant plasma fasting insulin levels. Additionally, the resulting decrease in hepatic energy status activates AMPK (AMP-activated protein kinase), a cellular metabolic sensor, having action on hepatic gluconeogenesis. It depicted marvelous non-glycemic related effects. The drug because of positive charge, can only partially cross the plasma membrane by passive diffusion. Its intracellular pathways are mediated by different isomers of organic cation transporters (OCT 1 for liver tissues and OCT 2 in the kidneys). These effects include modulation of different points of cancer timeline, weight reduction, cardiovascular health, thyroid diseases, polycystic ovaries disease and many other medical conditions. The aim of this review is to familiarize the effects of metformin in non-diabetes related medical disorders, advances in our understanding of this drug and its pathways in health and diseases.

Keywords: metformin, anti-proliferative, AMPK, mTOR, endothelium, insulin resistance

1. Introduction

History of metformin is linked to Galega officinalis (also known as goat's rue), a traditional herbal medicine in Europe, found to be rich in guanidine, which, in 1918, was shown to lower blood glucose. Guanidine derivatives, including metformin, were synthesized and some (not metformin) were used to treat diabetes in the 1920s and 1930s but were discontinued due to toxicity. Metformin was rediscovered in the search for antimalarial agents in 1940s. It proved to be useful in clinical cases to treat influenza when it had also shown to lower blood glucose. This property was pursued by the French physician Jean Sterne, who first reported the use of metformin to treat diabetes in 1957.

Metformin is under use over 65 years worldwide. The data has shown beneficial effects of the drug on obesity, PCOS, fatty liver disease, cardiovascular dysfunction as anti-oxidant and on inflammation, besides its use in pre diabetic and diabetic subjects. Moreover, drug has ardent usefulness in various malignant conditions, Alzheimer's disease and dementias. The literature is also rich on use of metformin in diabetic and non-diabetic related effects on endocrinal disorders, especially on thyroid and different malignant conditions. The present review is focused on these alternate non-diabetic uses of metformin.

2. Metformin structure and pharmacology

Metformin is a plant based medicinal product a synthetic guanidine with two coupled molecules with loss of ammonia, hence named biguanide with additional substitution. Metformin structure is shown below:

Metformin

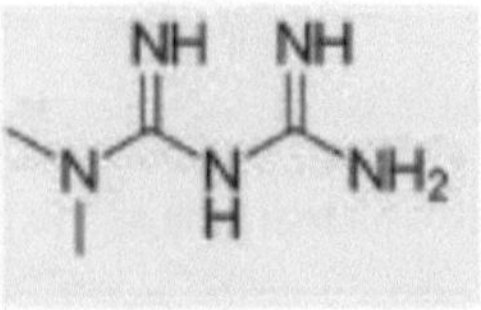

Metformin is conjugate base, a member of the class of guanidines that is biguanide the carrying two methyl substituents at position 1. It has a role as a hypoglycemic agent, a xenobiotic, an environmental contaminant and a gero protector. It derives from a biguanide.

Galega or guanidine is extracted from herbal plant G. officinalis [1]. Attention was paid initially on guanidine itself. The drug proved too toxic for clinical use. The drug is mainly absorbed from upper intestine with bioavailability of around 50%. The plasma half-life ranges from 0.9 to 2.6 h varying with different formulations. The transportation into the cell is via organic transporter-3 (OCT 3 & OCT 1). The drug is excreted unchanged in urine. This oral medicine is mainly concentrated in liver, kidney and jejunum site [2]. Because of short half-life and low oral bioavailability GI tract upsets are often noticed with the therapy. This limitations have overcome by designing delivery system and development of novel formulations. The drug delivery system have been investigated to decrease the side effects, frequency of dosage and enhancing the effect of oral anti-diabetic drug. The interest with novel formulations with nanoparticles is expected to improve drug bioavailability, dosing, frequency and GI tract side effects. The process of nano particles in the optimized concentration and surface characteristics has generated a great potential offer for treatment of type 2 diabetic mellitus [3]. The rational development of nano skilled delivery system has been described in literature by many workers [4, 5]. Their objectives were to achieve specific advantages using apt nano size and surface modifications of the particles to improve the target delivery of the drug to any compartment of the body at cellular and subcellular levels. Improving therapeutic potentials are the main goals of this drug delivery system in their researches [5].

Around 120 million people worldwide are using the drug as antihyperglycemic agent, without much having overt hypoglycemic episodes. In human beings, the drug molecules works at 2 levels: at liver level and at peripheral tissues.

The process is active through AMPK (adenosine monophosphate protein kinase) as cell regulatory mechanism. In humans, AMPK is essential for metabolism of glucose and fatty acids by downsizing glucose output from the liver, reducing gluconeogenesis and fatty acid synthesis in the liver. AMPK is essential for enhancing glucose uptake and fatty acid oxidation in peripheral muscles. The beneficial effects are seen on multiple organ system. Mitochondrial metabolism is also found altered by metformin which helps in reduction in gluconeogenesis by down regulation. The drug mechanism has tumor modulation as prerogative role as adjunct therapy in cancer [6]. Metformin also inhibits GI uptake of carbohydrates, reduces leptin levels and results in augmentation of glucose like peptide on gut cells. At molecular level, metformin modulates Adenosine A1 receptors (ADORA 1) which are essential in the cellular energy cycle. The human colorectal cancer cells may remain energy deprived when ADORA 1 are downregulated with resultant apoptosis [6].

The certain authorities have commented that drug probably does not directly activate AMPK and LKB1gene. LKB1 gene is tumor suppressor gene {Serine/threonine kinase 11 (STK11) also known as **liver kinase B1** (LKB1)}. The drug does not influence the phosphorylation of AMPK by LKB1 in a cell free assay [7].

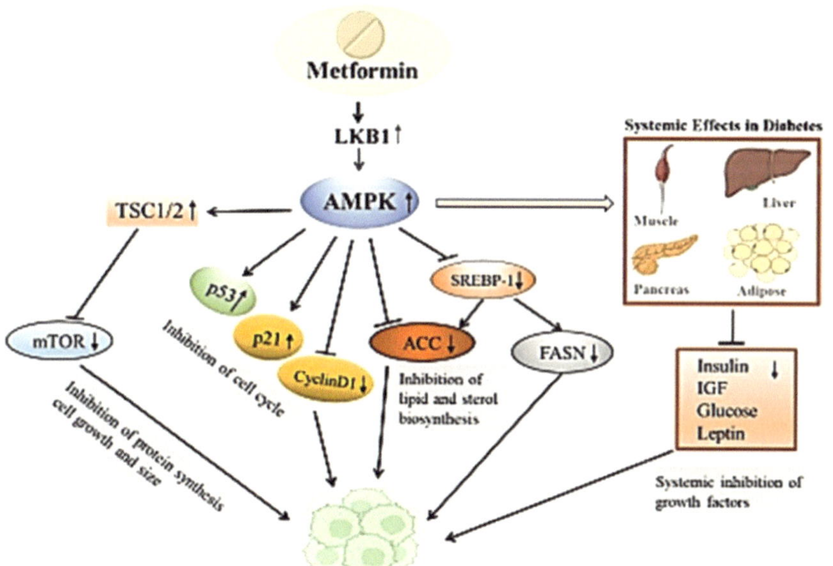

Figure 1.
Mechanism of action of metformin. Metformin activates AMPK through its effect on mitochondria. Growth inhibition include mTOR activity resulting in inhibition of protein synthesis and cell growth. AMPK activation also enhances p53 and p21 along with inhibition of cyclin D1. These small molecules exhibit divers' biological activities with inhibition of cell cycle. Inhibition of lipid and sterol biosynthesis pathway wide inhibition of sterol regulatory element – binding protein-1c (SREBP 1) and downregulation of fatty acid synthase. Inhibition of CoA carboxylase (ECC) influences tumor suppression. Source: Pharmaceuticals 2022, 15, 442. DOI: 10.3390/ph15040442.

Metformin activates AMPK through its effect on mitochondria. Growth inhibition include mTOR activity resulting in inhibition of protein synthesis and cell growth. AMPK activation also enhances p53 and p21 along with inhibition of cyclin D1. These small molecules exhibit diverse biological activities with inhibition of cell cycle. Inhibition of lipid and sterol biosynthesis pathway wide inhibition of sterol regulatory element – binding protein-1c (SREBP 1) and down regulation of fatty acid synthase. Inhibition of CO-A carboxylase (ECC) influences tumor suppression. The main mechanism of action of metformin and cancer is summarized in **Figure 1**. (Adopted from Chow Elaine and colleagues) [8].

3. Multifaceted impact of metformin

3.1 Antioxidant activity

The exact privileged mechanism is yet unclear. The antioxidant effect includes decreased gluconeogenesis and activation of AMPK system, upregulation of protein to fat and beta cell oxidation that lead to increase in the fatty acid metabolism and beta oxidation in fatty tissue [9]. A healthy heart obtains 60–90% energy for oxidative phosphorylation from fatty acid oxidation, whereas a failing heart has a balance for increase the glucose uptake and utilization [10]. The utilization of fatty acids use more oxygen per unit of ATP than the generated glucose which may improve ventricular performance. The drug also normalized non-esterified fatty acids, suggesting metabolic adaptation with use of the drug, as the drug modifies cardiac lipid/glucose oxidation ratio. Further, metformin action on cardiomyocytes attenuates the production of pro-apoptotic proteins, increase in anti-apoptotic proteins that reduce the percentage of apoptotic cardiomyocytes [11]. The studies with support of AMPK on endothelial functions revealed beneficial effects on it, suppressing oxidative stress in endothelial cell [12]. Thus, findings related to oxidative stress in endothelial cells, cardiomyocytes functionality and production of radical oxidative substrates (ROS) are inhibited by metformin which helps in preventing endothelial dysfunction, atherogenesis and improves myocardial dysfunction. Metformin is avoided in patient with heart failure because of risk of lactic acidosis. Currently, this contraindication weighs insignificance in literature [13]. Eurich and coworkers in 2011, indeed suggested that metformin alone or in combination with sulphonylurea reduce both the mortality and morbidity of type 2 diabetic patients with heart failure in comparison with Sulphonylurea as monotherapy [14].

3.2 Endothelial function and anti-inflammatory agent

The mechanism of metformin on endothelial function is unclear. However, endothelial function modulation was suggested in acquiring insulin resistance improvement. Endothelial dysfunctions are chiefly observed in diabetic and patients of ischemic heart disease [15]. The results of metformin as anti-inflammatory agent is controversial [16]. Metformin inhibits nuclear factor kappa B (NF-kB) by down regulating inflammatory responses. The factor NF-kB, a protein transcription factor is also a regulator of innate immunity.

3.3 Obesity and hormonal imbalances

It is argued by many researchers that weight reduction by metformin per say is owing to diabetic related medications rather the drug itself. The weight changes are evidently observed with impaired glucose tolerance unlike diabetics without obesity where in the drug failed to reduce the weight significantly [17]. Others elaborated the reasons for reduction in weight with metformin which are (1) reduction in leptin levels, (2) augmentation of glucagon like peptide one effects on fatty tissues, (3) reduction in carbohydrates uptake by the gut [18]. Metformin induced reduction in hepatic lipid content is consistent with increase in fatty acid oxidation and inhibition of lipogenesis mediated through AMPK activation [19].

3.4 PCOS (polycystic ovarian syndrome)

It is now recognized that insulin resistance, is a common feature of PCOS. The disorder affects at least 5–15% of reproductive age women. Pharmacological option in PCOS and insulin resistance with insulin sensitizer are being proposed. Metformin medications increased ovulation, reduce serum androgen levels [20].

The beneficial effects of metformin are based on production of excess insulin or ovarian effects. Insulin directly stimulates enzymes in ovary such as cytochrome P_{450}, 3beta SHD (3 beta hydroxysteroids) by improving insulin sensitivity by CYP 17 (cytochrome P450) activity, inhibits androstenedione effects on theta cells, reduces factors such as endometrial androgen receptor expression - factors with high risk of abortion. The observations have clinical significance that the use of metformin in an overweight PCOS patient would be fruitful. Metformin has been shown to reduce risks of abortion in PCOS in pregnancy.

3.5 Thyroid gland function

Metformin is considered a cornerstone of type 2 diabetes medication umbrella. Many prospective and retrospective studies have shown that serum TSH levels in hypothyroid patients decreased in response to metformin therapy and increased again when metformin was withdrawn [21]. Relevant changes were not observed in serum thyroxine (T4), triiodothyronine (T3) levels. In a study, by Cappali et al. [22] in 2009 that diabetic patient on metformin, had significant decline levels of TSH, but T4, T3 remained unchanged for 1 year. The changes were also noticed in group with already existing hypothyroidism on medication irrespective of metformin therapy. Following this initial findings a number of studies that were performed elucidated various mechanisms of the drug on TSH level. Metformin was shown to have a lowering effect on TSH level. Metformin likely affects thyroid function through peripheral conversion of thyroxine to triiodothyronine [23] when TSH value was higher than 2.98 mU/L, whereas the opposite effect was seen on individual having serum TSH level lower than 2.98 mU/L. The thyrotropin effect was not observed in hyperthyroid subjects with type 2 diabetes [24].

Use of metformin is hypothesized to change the affinity of thyroid hormones to increase the dopaminergic tone or induce activation of TSH receptors [21].

Metformin is also found to modulate hypothalamic pituitary thyroid axis at the level of peripheral tissues. The observations indicated that metformin treatment could have an impact on thyrotropin function in hypothyroid patient in apart associated with alterations in dopaminergic regulation of thyrotropin secretion.

Duntas et al. [25] suggested that metformin is proved to have inhibitory effect on AMPK activity in hypothalamus. Clinical studies under taken by Al-Alu-Si 2015 [26], concluded that levothyroxine absorption remains unchanged by concomitant metformin. TSH suppression effect of metformin may be useful in clinical hyperthyroidism. However, complexity exist for monitoring thyroid function status in diabetic patient on metformin. The depressed TSH level may provide false reassurance in decreasing T4 (levothyroxine) dosage with low TSH level. The proper interpretation of thyroid functions is mandatory in patients receiving metformin therapy in diabetes.

3.6 Central nervous system

Metformin effect on nervous system is also puzzling. In Alzheimer's disease, there is remarkable progressive insulin resistance of the brain cells leading to formation of amyloid cells. The disease is unofficially considered as type-3 diabetes. The brain cells here are dependent on glucose for survival and have low antioxidant enzyme contents as a result of oxidative injuries. Activation of AMPK pathway play a vital role in reducing insulin resistance and oxidative stress. The drug metformin is known to activate AMPK thus, partially could have a protective role in Alzheimer's disease and others oxidative distress related neurological disorders. Metformin also plays a pivotal role in breaking the cycle of permeability transition protein release in the mitochondria. By virtue of drug effect, metformin in the mitochondria, plays a role in this cascade with resultant delay in the program of cell death [27]. The drug metformin influences and reduces neuro inflammatory status along with glucose metabolism leading to protein dephosphorylation, acts as an anti-oxidant and helps reducing neuro inflammation and degeneration (**Figure 2**).

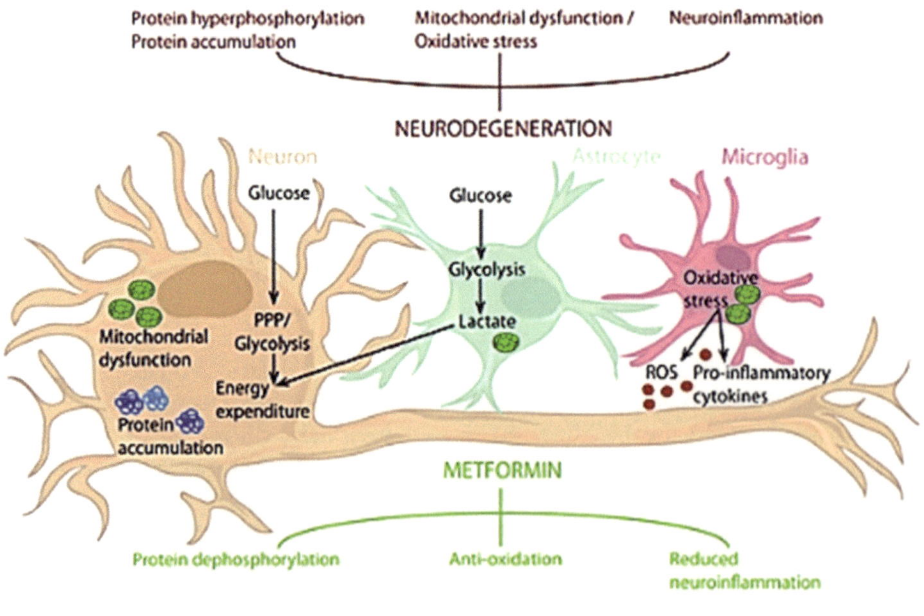

Figure 2.
Metformin effects in neuron. It shows metformin counteraction protein hyperphosphorylation, oxidative stress and neuro inflammation, neuro fibrillary tangles, processes known to drive neural loss. The drug metformin influence neuro inflammatory status along with glucose metabolism leading to protein dephosphorylation, as an anti-oxidant and reducing neuro inflammation. Source: (https://www.researchgate.net/figure/Metformins-potential-as-a-neuroprotective-agent-Metformin-can-counteract-protein).

3.7 Anti-retroviral agents

HIV treatments lead to metabolic consequences as insulin resistance, dysregulation of glucose metabolism, dyslipidemia, and lipodystrophy in 80% of subjects as side effects of medication. Metformin as an adjunct therapy, diet and exercise effectively prevent these consequences by improving visceral fat distribution, reduces risk of insulin insensitivity, dyslipidemia, weight gain, hyperglycemia and endothelial dysfunctions.

3.8 Renal cancer

AMPK which suppresses the cell proliferation. AMPK pathway subsequently lead to inhibition of mTOR that is responsible for cell growth. mTOR the mammalian/mechanistic target of rapamycin is a kinase that in humans is encoded of MTOR gene. mTOR pathway is involved in number of important physiological functions including cell growth, cell proliferation, metabolism and protein synthesis. Inhibition of mTOR vide AMPK pathway is responsible for anti-proliferative effect. Metformin is also known to inhibit mTOR independently of AMPK pathway, making the outcome more effective in controlling the proliferation of cell growth. Metformin not only prevents phosphorylation of mTORc1 complex component but also inhibits phosphorylation of AKT, a mTORc2 substrate which is beneficial in the treatment of cancer.

3.9 COVID19

Metformin blocks the viruses from binding the host receptors ACE2. Other effects of metformin are AKT inhibition, AMPK activation, inhibition of mTOR activity there by suppressing virus – host protein interaction. The drug also inhibits mitochondrial generation of ROS which leads to rising intracellular calcium and subsequent release of pro-inflammatory cytokines (IL1, IL6, TNF alpha and IL beta). In COVID 19 infection, the drug metformin increases insulin sensitivity that modify endosomal pH and reduces viral replications and maturation. ACE2 downregulation by SARS Co-2 is prevented by metformin. This drug mediated increase levels of ACE2 and phosphorylation of ACE2 subsequently regulates RAAS and offers cardiopulmonary protection.

4. Therapeutic applications of metformin

4.1 Cancer

The large number of cohort studies have confirmed the significance of associated diabetes mellitus with increased risk of cancer affecting pancreas, kidney, prostate, colon and breast. This increased risk is attributed to persistently elevated plasma glucose and plasma insulin levels. Insulin resistance, hyperinsulinemia that might promote carcinogenesis, directly or indirectly increasing levels of insulin-like growth factor (IGF) (formerly called somatomedin) that functions primarily to stimulate growth. However, that also possess some ability to decrease blood glucose levels and inflammatory process [28].

Metformin therapy in these malignant cases were associated with relative reduce risk of cancer and cancer mortality in diabetic patient [29]. These observations are consistently seen with *in vitro* and *invivo* studies revealing anti-proliferative action of metformin on various cancer lines [30].

4.1.1 Breast cancer

As mentioned previously, the action of metformin is having direct effect on AMPK that when occurs, lowers the ATP ratio in cells resulting in stimulating AMPK pathway for regularizing energy homeostasis. Excess energy, in turn will signal the need to decrease the energy consumption. Thus, resulting cytotoxic effects are met with inhibition of cell growth and proliferation of breast tissue. Further, Metformin is known to exert an indirect effect on cells by lowering insulin levels and decreasing PI3k pathway, inhibiting cell growth and proliferation. PI3k signaling pathway stimulates the cells for proliferation and growth, simultaneously inhibiting cell apoptosis. It is an enzyme that transmit signal in cells that helps to control the cell growth. Some tumors have higher level than normal of PI3k (PI3 kinase). By inhibiting this enzyme, PI3k inhibitors cause cell death and inhibit the proliferation of malignant cell. Iliopoulos and coworkers [31] in 2011, suggested the need of higher dosage of metformin (1.5–2.5 g) to attain anti-neoplastic effect [31].

4.1.2 Liver cancer

Lack of well-designed trials on the subject, reserves the outcome of metformin use in liver cancer. However, in metaanalysis compiled by zhang and colleagues concluded that metformin appears playing a role in reducing liver cancer risk in type 2 DM [32]. More well designed trials would be needed to evaluate this point.

4.1.3 Pancreatic cancer

Many trials have assessed possible link between type 2 diabetic and pancreatic cancer. The study by Huxley et al. [33] 2005, noticed in their study a higher risk of pancreatic cancer development in diabetic subjects who are having short duration of illness. Yet another study revealed to significantly lower risk of mortality in patients with pancreatic cancer who used metformin [34]. More further studies needed to consolidate this conclusion.

4.1.4 Endometrial cancer

A large numbers of studies had explained the improvement of overall survival in patient with advanced endometrial cancer taking metformin. Studied patients were either diabetic or non-diabetic [35, 36]. Metformin's role in recurrence of endometrial cancer as remained unclear. Prospective study under taken by Soliman et al. in 2016 in newly diagnosed endometrial cancer, demonstrated the reduction in serum molecular markers of cancer who were using metformin in a week's period [36]. It is also described that mechanism of metformin in tumor cell is vide FOXO 1 pathway involvement. FOXO family is a subclass of fork head transcription factors. The pathway is responsible for regulating the expression of gene in the cellular physiological events including apoptosis, cell cycling control, glucose metabolism, oxidative stress resistance etc. It was also revealed that providing a AMPK inhibition in the FOXO 1 pathway by injecting silencing RNA for FOXO 1 in endometrial cell, subsequently eradicated anti-proliferative effects of metformin. The observation bears strong therapeutic implication [37, 38]. The proposed scheme for the antiproliferative mechanism of metformin in estrogen-dependent endometrial cancer (EC) cells is shown in **Figure 3** (Source: [39]).

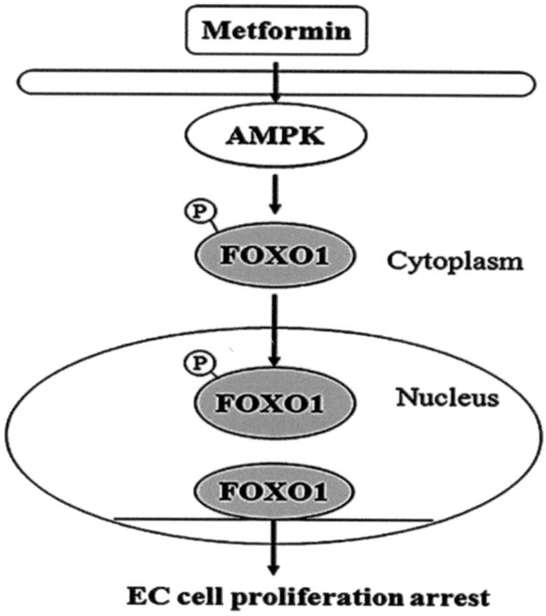

Figure 3.
Proposed scheme for the antiproliferative mechanism of metformin in estrogen-dependent endometrial cancer (EC) cells. Metformin activates AMPK/human forkhead FOXO1 –P in the cytoplasm thus decreasing phosphorylation (P) of FOXO1 protein. There by organizing RE localisation of FOXO1 protein from cytoplasm to nucleus with enhance FOXO1 activity. FOXO1 function contributes to increased efficacy of metformin therapy against EC-novel mechanism of metformin as anti-neoplastic. Findings are supportive for prostate cervical cancer.

4.1.5 Cervical cancer

Limited data is available on this subject. Xiao et al. 2012 [40] examined metformin dynamics in these cancer cells with focus on LKB1. Cell lines were either responsive to metformin or remained non-responsive to metformin. The cell lines which are responsive to metformin stimulate AMPK via LKB1 and prevents mTOR. Nonresponsive cell to metformin were void of LKB1. LKB1 gene also known as STK 1 gene, provides instruction for making enzyme called serine/threonine kinase 1. This enzyme is a tumor suppresser that helps the cells in growing and its division rapidly. Metformin also suppress other cell lines of cervical cancer cell viz. C33A, ME180. Metformin may, Therefore, have an adjuvant role especially in such cervical cancer having presence of LKB1 cell line. C33A is an epithelial cell line isolated from cervix of uterine cancer patient. Herein, arginine to cystine substitution takes place at codon 273.

4.1.6 Lung cancer

Poor association are shown between use of metformin and lung cancer [41]. A retrospective cohort study by wink et al. [42] had concluded that patients of diabetics on metformin and with locally advanced non-small cell (NSCL) cancer where having less chances of disease progression and metastasis, than those who were not kept on metformin [42].

4.1.7 Colorectal cancer

Diabetic patients are shown to have lower risk of colorectal carcinoma when treated with metformin. Besides metformin is having the ability to lower the risk of colorectal cancer, improvement and survival in such patients [43–45].

4.1.8 Renal cancer

Metformin is a common therapeutic agent with anti-tumor activity in various cancer types. However, its use remains controversial in renal cell carcinoma. Adjunct metformin treatment in RCC (renal cell carcinoma) lead to activation of. In RCC additional, anti-proliferative effects are also achieved by suppression of cyclin D gene responsible for cell proliferation and cell growth [46]. Metformin is also able to prevent renal cell carcinoma by incorporating the regulation of gene miR-26a, which will inhibit cyclin D1 expression- a factor incumbent for the cell growth. mTORc1and c2 promote the cell growth by inducing and inhibiting anabolic and catabolic processes respectively and drives the cell cycle progression. In clinical practice, metformin has shown insignificant association in preventing the recurrences of RCC after its resection [47].

4.2 COVID19

After the emergence in late December 2019, it was observed by many workers, that diabetic individuals were at high risk of COVID 19 infection and its associated complications. Interestingly, diabetic COVID 19 patients had more adverse outcome while on insulin when compared to those who were on metformin. Metformin treatment correlated with significant reduction in disease severity and mortality in such cases. Excellent review on the subject is published by Varghese E and colleagues in 2021 [48]. The drug has its role as anti-oxidant, anti-inflammatory, immunomodulator, and protective effects on vasculature and endothelial functions, already discussed earlier in the text. It is noteworthy to mention that ACE2 receptor is expressed in various organs viz. brain, heart, lung, intestine, kidney, liver, vasculature and adipose tissues making them targets for COVID infections. Diabetes has increased expression of ACE2 in various tissues hence leading to increase in viral load Metformin provides protection metabolically and reduces complications related to immune response and thrombotic events. Metformin in COVID 19 be judiciously used with conditions such as renal failure, diabetic ketoacidosis and severely ill patients.

5. Conclusion

Despite newer advances made for oral hypoglycemic agents metformin remains as main agent under diabetic umbrella. The drug has effectively demonstrated to possess anti-tumor activity of value in varied cancer subjects. The main effect of drug is to decrease hepatic glucose production by mitochondrial respiratory chain complex resulting in transient decline in cellular energy status that promotes the activation of AMPK, a well-known cellular sensor. There are multiple molecular mechanisms proposed about metformin with protective properties in diabetic and non-diabetic users. Morewider researches with their clinical implications still are awaiting for metformin use as an adjunct therapy in various cancer subjects.

6. Future perspective

Well-designed human and animal researches are needed to confirm the benefits of drugs in as anti-inflammatory agent, anti-proliferative agent in various inflammatory and malignant disorders. Nanoparicles/microbubbles generated drug for treatment of diabetes mellitus has great potential but needs further researches with specific attention to optimized concentration. Extensive physiologic and biochemical studies are still required to identify indirect targets influenced by relatively limited number of direct targets.

7. Recommendations

Metformin is currently recommend as first line glucose lowering drug in type 2 diabetes mellitus. Molecular studies though highlight the knowledge gap in areas of unearth needs, However, neo clinical and mechanistic studies on metformin and its usefulness on central nervous system, infections and cancers are warranted with new insight into its therapeutic value beyond boundaries of diabetes.

Author details

Shafaat Husain Talib*, Umar Quadri, Sachin Patel and Pranita Barapatre
Department of Medicine, MGM Medical College, Aurangabad, India

*Address all correspondence to: sftalib@gmail.com

References

[1] Bailey CJ. Metformin: Historical overview. Diabetologia. 2017;**60**: 1566-1576

[2] Bailey CJ, Wilcock C, Scarpello JH. Metformin and the intestine. Diabetologia. 2008;**51**:1552-1553

[3] Cesur S, Cam ME, Sayın FS, et al. Metformin-Loaded Polymer-aq3Based Microbubbles/ Nanoparticles Generated for the Treatment of Type 2 Diabetes Mellitus. 2021. Langmuir 2022;**38**(17):5040-5051

[4] Cafferata EA, Alvarez C, Diaz KT, Maureira M, Monasterio G, GonzálezFE.Multifunctionalnanocarriers for the treatmentof periodontitis: Immunomodulatory, antimicrobial, and regenerative strategies. Oral Diseases. 2019;**25**(8):1866-1878

[5] Taghipour YD, Bahramsoltani R, Marques AM, Naseri R, Rahimi R, Haratipour P, et al. A systematic review of nano formulation of natural products for the treatment of inflammatory bowel disease: Drug delivery and pharmacological targets. Daru. 2018;**26**(2):229-239

[6] Lan B, Zhang J, Zhang P, Zhang W, Yang S, Lu D, et al. Metformin suppresses CRC growth by inducing apoptosis via ADORA1. Frontiers in Bioscience. 2017;**22**:248-257

[7] Hardie DG. Neither LKB1 nor AMPK are the direct targets of metformin. Gastroenterology. 2006;**131**:973

[8] de Sousa A, Pereira BF, Laura M, de Souza L, da Silva-Junior AA, et al. Invitro-in vivo availability of metformin hydrochloride-PLGA nanoparticles in diabetic rats in a periodontal disease experimental model. Pharmaceutical Biology. 2021;**59**(1):1574-1582. DOI: 10.1080/13880209.2021.2002369

[9] Anedda A, Rial E, Gonzalez-Barroso MM. Metformin induces oxidative stress in white adipocytes and raises uncoupling protein 2 levels. The Journal of Endocrinology. 2008;**199**(1):33-40

[10] Lopaschuk GD. Optimizing cardiac fatty acid and glucose metabolism as an approach to treating heart failure. Seminars in Cardiothoracic and Vascular Anesthesia. 2006;**10**:228-230

[11] Yeh CH, Chen TP, Wang YC, Lin YM, Fang SW. AMP-activated protein kinase activation during cardioplegia-induced hypoxia/reoxygenation injury attenuates cardiomyocytic apoptosis via reduction of endoplasmic reticulum stress. Mediators of Inflammation. 2010;**2010**:130636

[12] Zou MH, Wu Y. AMP-activated protein kinase activation as a strategy for protecting vascular endothelial function. Clinical and Experimental Pharmacology & Physiology. 2008;**35**:535-545

[13] Hurana R, Malik IS. Metformin: Safety in cardiac patients. Heart. 2010;**96**:99-102

[14] Eurich DT, Majumdar SR, McAlister FA, Tsuyuki RT, Johnson JA. Improved clinical outcomes associated with metformin in patients with diabetes and heart failure. Diabetes Care. 2005;**28**:2345-2351

[15] VitaleC,MercuroG,CornoldiA,FiniM, Volterrani M, Rosano GM. Metformin improves endothelial function in patients

with metabolic syndrome. Journal of Internal Medicine. 2005;**258**(3):250-256

[16] Haffner S, Temprosa M, Crandall J, Fowler S, Goldberg R, Horton E, et al. Intensive lifestyle intervention or metformin on inflammation and coagulation in participants with impaired glucose tolerance. Diabetes. 2005;**54**(5):1566-1572

[17] Lily M, Godwin M. Treating prediabetes with metformin: Systematic review and meta-analysis. Canadian Family Physician. 2009;**55**(4):363-369

[18] Glueck CJ, Fontaine RN, Wang P, Subbiah MT, Weber K, Illig E, et al. Metformin reduces weight, centripetal obesity, insulin, leptin, and low-density lipoprotein cholesterol in nondiabetic, morbidly obese subjects with body mass index greater than 30. Metabolism. 2001;**50**(7):856-861

[19] Zhou G, Myers R, Li Y, Chen Y, Shen X, Melody J, et al. Role of AMP-activated protein kinase in mechanism of metformin action. The Journal of Clinical Investigation. 2001;**108**:1167-1174

[20] Tang T, Lord JM, Norman RJ, Yasmin E, Balen AH. Insulin-sensitising drugs (metformin, rosiglitazone, pioglitazone, D-chiro-inositol) for women with polycystic ovary syndrome, oligo amenorrhoea and subfertility. The Cochrane Database of Systematic Reviews. 2009;(4):CD003053

[21] Vigersky RA, Filmore-Nassar A, Glass AR. Thyrotropin suppression by metformin. The Journal of Clinical Endocrinology and Metabolism. 2006;**91**(1):225-227

[22] Cappelli C, Rotondi M, Pirola I, Agosti B, Gandossi E, Valentini U. TSH-lowering effect of metformin in type 2 diabetic patients: Differences between euthyroid, untreated hypothyroid, and euthyroid on L-T4 therapy patients. Diabetes Care. 2009;**32**:1589-1590

[23] Vella S, Cachia MJ, Vassallo J. The effects of metformin on thyroid function. Poster presentation at the spring meeting of the Scottish Society for Experimental Medicine. (Aberdeen, 29th May, 2009)

[24] Krysiak R, Okopien B. Thyrotropin-lowering effect of metformin in a patient with resistance to thyroid hormone. Clinical Endocrinology. 2011;**75**:404-406

[25] Isidro ML, Penin MA, Nemina R, Cordido F. Metformin reduces thyrotropin levels in obese, diabetic women with primary hypothyroidism on thyroxine replacement therapy. Endocrine. 2007;**32**(1):79-82

[26] Meng X, Xu S, Chen G et al. Metformin and thyroid disease. Journal of Endocrinology. 2017;**233**(1):R43-R51

[27] van der Heide LP, Ramakers GM, Smidt MP. Insulin signaling in the central nervous system: Learning to survive. Progress in Neurobiology. 2006;**79**(4):205-221

[28] Jalving M, Gietema JA, Lefrandt JD, de Jong S, Reyners AK, Gans RO, et al. Metformin: Taking away the candy for cancer? European Journal of Cancer. 2010;**46**:2369-2380

[29] Bowker SL, Yasui Y, Veugelers P, Johnson JA. Glucose-lowering agents and cancer mortality rates in type 2 diabetes: Assessing effects of time-varying exposure. Diabetologia. 2010;**53**:1631-1637

[30] Ben Sahra I, Le Marchand-Brustel Y, Tanti JF, Bost F. Metformin in cancer therapy: A new perspective for an old antidiabetic drug? Molecular Cancer Therapeutics. 2010;**9**:1092-1099

[31] Iliopoulos D, Hirsch HA, Struhl K. Metformin decreases the dose of chemotherapy for prolonging tumor remission in mouse xenografts involving multiple cancer cell types. Cancer Research. 2011;**71**(9):3196-3201

[32] Zhang ZJ, Zheng ZJ, Shi R, Su Q, Jiang Q, Kip KE. Metformin for liver cancer prevention in patients with type 2 diabetes: A systematic review and meta-analysis. The Journal of Clinical Endocrinology and Metabolism. 2012;**97**(7):2347-2353

[33] Huxley R, Ansary-Moghaddam A, Berrington de Gonzalez A, Barzi F, Woodward M. Type-II diabetes and pancreatic cancer: A meta-analysis of 36 studies. British Journal of Cancer. 2005;**92**(11):2076-2083

[34] Cerullo M, Gani F, Chen SY, Canner J, Pawlik TM. Metformin use is associated with improved survival in patients undergoing resection for pancreatic cancer. Journal of Gastrointestinal Surgery. 2016;**20**(9):1572-1580

[35] Ko EM, Walter P, Jackson A, Clark L, Franasiak J, Bolac C, et al. Metformin is associated with improved survival in endometrial cancer. Gynecologic Oncology. 2014;**132**(2):438-442

[36] Soliman PT, Zhang Q, Broaddus RR, Westin SN, Iglesias D, Munsell MF, et al. Prospective evaluation of the molecular effects of metformin on the endometrium in women with newly diagnosed endometrial cancer: A window of opportunity study. Gynecologic Oncology. 2016;**143**(3):466-471

[37] Zou J, Hong L, Luo C, Li Z, Zhu Y, Huang T, et al. Metformin inhibits estrogen-dependent endometrial cancer cell growth by activating the AMPK-FOXO1 signal pathway. Cancer Science. 2016;**107**(12):1806-1817

[38] Li R, Erdamar S, Dai H, et al. Forkhead protein FKHR and its phosphorylated form p-FKHR in human prostate cancer. Human Pathology. 2007;**38**:1501-1507

[39] Zhang B, Gui LS, Zhao XL, Zhu LL, Li QW. FOXO1 is a tumor suppressor in cervical cancer. Genetics and Molecular Research. 2015;**14**:6605-6616

[40] Xiao X, He Q, Lu C, Werle KD, Zhao RX, Chen J, et al. Metformin impairs the growth of liver kinase B1-intact cervical cancer cells. Gynecologic Oncology. 2012;**127**(1):249-255

[41] Sakoda LC, Ferrara A, Achacoso NS, Peng T, Ehrlich SF, Quesenberry CP, et al. Metformin use and lung cancer risk in patients with diabetes. Cancer Prevention Research (Philadelphia, Pa.). 2015;**8**(2):174-179

[42] Wink KC, Belderbos JS, Dieleman EM, Rossi M, Rasch CR, Damhuis RA, et al. Improved progression free survival for patients with diabetes and locally advanced non-small cell lung cancer (NSCLC) using metformin during concurrent chemoradiotherapy. Radiotherapy and Oncology. 2016;**118**(3):453-459

[43] He XK, Su TT, Si JM, Sun LM. Metformin is associated with slightly reduced risk of colorectal cancer and moderate survival benefits in diabetes mellitus: A meta-analysis. Medicine (Baltimore). 2016;**95**(7):e2749. pp. 1-10

[44] Singh S, Singh H, Singh PP, Murad MH, Limburg PJ. Antidiabetic medications and the risk of colorectal cancer in patients with diabetes mellitus: A systematic review and meta-analysis. Cancer Epidemiology, Biomarkers & Prevention. 2013;**22**(12):2258-2268

[45] Lee JH, Jeon SM, Hong SP, Cheon JH, Kim TI, Kim WH. Metformin use is

associated with a decreased incidence of colorectal adenomas in diabetic patients with previous colorectal cancer. Digestive and Liver Disease. 2012;**44**(12):1042-1047

[46] Liu J, Li M, Song B, Jia C, Zhang L, Bai X, et al. Metformin inhibits renal cell carcinoma in vitro and in vivo xenograft. Urologic Oncology. 2013;**31**(2):264-270

[47] Cerezo M, Tichet M, Abbe P, et al. Metformin blocks melanoma invasion and metastasis development in AMPK/p53-dependent manner. Molecular Cancer Therapeutics. 2013;**12**(8):1605-1615

[48] Varghese E, Samuel SM, Liskova A, Kubatka P, Büsselberg D. Diabetes and coronavirus (SARS-CoV-2): Molecular mechanism of Metformin intervention and the scientific basis of drug repurposing. PLOS Pathogens. 2021;**17**(6):e1009634. pp.1-20